D0467317

REACHING OUT IN FAMILY THERAPY

Reaching Out in Family Therapy

Home-Based, School, and Community Interventions

NANCY BOYD-FRANKLIN
BRENNA HAFER BRY

THE GUILFORD PRESS
New York   London

© 2000 The Guilford Press
A Division of Guilford Publications, Inc.
72 Spring Street, New York, NY 10012
www.guilford.com

Printed in the United States of America

This book is printed on acid-free paper.

Last digit is print number: 9   8   7   6   5   4   3   2   1

Library of Congress Cataloging-in-Publication Data is available from the Publisher.

ISBN 1-57230-519-3

To A. J.,
for all of his love and support.
—N. B. F.

To Perry and Ethel Hafer,
who first showed me how to reach out.
—B. H. B.

About the Authors

Nancy Boyd-Franklin, PhD, is an African American family therapist and Professor in the Graduate School of Applied and Professional Psychology at Rutgers University. She is the author of *Black Families in Therapy: A Multisystems Approach* (Guilford Press, 1989) and coeditor of *Children, Families, and HIV/AIDS: Psychosocial and Therapeutic Issues* (Guilford Press, 1995). An internationally recognized lecturer and author, Dr. Boyd-Franklin has written numerous articles on issues such as ethnicity and family therapy, the treatment of African American families, extended family issues, spirituality and religion, home-based family therapy, group therapy for Black women, HIV and AIDS, parent and family support groups, community empowerment, and the multisystems model.

Brenna Hafer Bry, PhD, is Professor of Clinical Psychology in the Graduate School of Applied and Professional Psychology at Rutgers University, and has over 25 years of experience in home-based family, school, and community interventions and research. Dr. Bry has devoted her career to identifying at-risk youth and developing and evaluating early intervention programs for them and their families. One of her original school-based interventions recently was renamed the Behavioral Monitoring and Reinforcement Program and designated an "effective strategy" by the U.S. Department of Education's Safe and Drug Free Schools Program.

Preface

We have felt for some time the need in our field for a book that focuses on outreach to children, adolescents, and their families. To help fill this need, we have written this book, which emphasizes "reaching out" in home-based family therapy, in the schools, and in the community. Our goal is to provide a resource for practitioners of all kinds: family therapists, psychologists, social workers, physicians, nurses, counselors, teachers and guidance counselors, child welfare workers, and those working in the juvenile justice and substance abuse fields. In order to be as inclusive as possible, we refer to practitioners throughout this book as family therapists, family workers, counselors, and clinicians. This book offers them helpful conceptualizations, effective strategies, relevant research, and multiple case examples.

Although we approach this work from different paths, we have found that we share a common approach: in order to achieve intervention goals, we involve not only the families but also outside systems that affect the families—schools, courts, welfare and child protection agencies, and churches. Many of the families we see face complex sociopolitical and socioeconomic realities such as racism, poverty, sexism, and the challenges associated with immigration. The multisystems, structural, and behavioral family therapy models provide theoretical frameworks that guide us in the proactive interventions we describe throughout this book. Our treatment strategies are designed to empower families and therapists to be more effective through a collaborative partnership.

We bring to this work many of the experiences of "frontline" clinical and preventive interventions, supervision, teaching, and training that we have had over the past 25 years. Nancy Boyd-Franklin began her training in structural family therapy at the Philadelphia Child Guidance Clinic. She was taught and influenced by the innovative work of Salvador Minuchin, Harry Aponte, Jay Haley, Braulio Montalvo, and Marianne Walters. Their early emphasis on working with families of the poor has impacted her work. Her interest in "extended" African American families and the issues facing other ethnic minority families has influenced the path she has chosen. The close collaboration she has shared with Monica McGoldrick and Paulette Hines has contributed significantly to her work on the influence of cultural and racial values in family therapy.

Brenna Hafer Bry is a cognitive-behavioral family therapist who was trained at Denison University by Irvin Wolf and at the University of Missouri in Columbia by Robert Daniel, Jacob Sines, David Premack, Mike Nawas, Eliot Hearst, and Janet Wollersheim. She has also appreciated over the years her collegial exchanges with Gerald Patterson and James Alexander. Her career has been devoted to identifying adolescents "at risk" for problems and developing and evaluating early intervention programs for them and their families. In addition to behavioral theory and feedback from practical experience, her empirical findings guide her work. Specifically, her research on risk factors for adolescent substance abuse, school failure, and juvenile delinquency convinces her of the necessity to both develop preventive approaches and include families in all interventions.

In recent years, we have both been increasingly aware that key family members often do not come into our clinics and schools. Our interest in home-based, school, and community interventions came from our desire to reach these individuals, who often have the power to bring about significant changes in their families. Our approach has continued to evolve—reinforced and elaborated by our clinical experience and research and by the work of the many therapists whom we supervise and train. For those readers who are actively involved in training practitioners, we hope that this book will provide ideas that will allow you to train and support therapists and other workers who are also "reaching out" to families.

Acknowledgments

We would like to give special thanks to all of those who have supported us in this work. First, we acknowledge our Dean, Sandra Harris, at the Graduate School of Applied and Professional Psychology, Rutgers University, and Dr. Stanley Messer, our Department Chair, for their encouragement and for the sabbatical leaves that have allowed us to devote time to this project. To Hazel Staloff, our editor and central word processor, we give thanks for the excellent quality of her work, her professional feedback, and ongoing encouragement.

At The Guilford Press, we are grateful for the contributions of Rochelle Serwator, our developmental editor, and Anna Nelson, who worked with us on the production of the book.

We would also like to give special thanks to our family members and close friends. Nancy thanks her husband, A. J. Franklin, and her mother, Regina Boyd, who read many drafts of the book and gave freely of their personal and professional expertise. She would also like to acknowledge her dear friend, Rosemary Allwood, for all of her input, clinical experience, and ongoing support. Finally, she gives special thanks to her son, Jay, and stepchildren and extended family, Deidre, Remi, Tunde, Debbie, Sergio, and Kaylan, for their love.

Brenna would like to express the deep admiration she feels for her children, David and Deborah, and thank them for all of the appreciation that they have shown her over the years. She would also like to remember fondly their father, Dr. Peter M. Bry, her late husband and partner in parenting.

We would both like to acknowledge our students, particularly Nancy Bloom, Tawn Smith Morris, and Carol Slechta, who coauthored chapters in this book. We would also like to thank all of the students in our classes who read early drafts of the book and gave us their excellent feedback.

Finally, together, we express admiration for and gratitude to the client families, from whom we continue to learn so much.

Contents

PART IV. RESEARCH AND SUPERVISION

PART I

OVERVIEW

CHAPTER 1

Introduction

This book draws from our collective experience of more than 25 years each of family therapy intervention and supervision. As family therapists, we have learned that it is vital to have a working model with which to organize interventions in complex situations. We see a broad range of families, each with difficult life circumstances and challenges. These include families at risk for substance abuse and/or domestic violence; families who are suspected of child abuse; families with young children, in which the adults are struggling with effective parenting; families with at-risk adolescents; and families with teenage parents or parents with HIV/AIDS.

The families we treat are composed of individuals with different needs and expectations, and of extended as well as nuclear family members. In some cultures, such as African American, West Indian, and Latino, close friends, neighbors, godparents, and members of the "church family" may also be considered members of the family.

Models that focus only on the individual, or only on the family, may be too constrained to provide an effective framework for intervention with these families. This is particularly true when one is working with poor families, in which different agencies and institutions often exercise a tremendous amount of power—including the ability to discontinue a family's financial support, medical care, or housing; to prosecute and/or incarcerate an individual; and to remove children from the home.

The approach we describe in this book is similar to traditional psychotherapy in some ways and different from it in many others. From traditional psychotherapeutic interventions, we have adopted weekly meetings with children, adolescents, and parents, and the process of talking as one method of influence. Beyond these aspects, our intervention is quite different. First, our approach is grounded in a *multisystems model.* And, second, *outreach* is an integral part of our work.

THE MULTISYSTEMS MODEL

We have combined our respective structural (Minuchin, 1974; Minuchin & Fishman, 1981; Minuchin & Nichols, 1993) and behavioral (Patterson, Reid, Jones, & Conger, 1975) family therapy approaches into a comprehensive "multisystems model." The multisystems model is a problem-solving approach that helps families with multiple problems to focus and prioritize their issues, and that allows clinicians to maximize the effectiveness of their interventions (Boyd-Franklin, 1989; Henggeler & Borduin, 1990; Henggeler, Schoenwald, Borduin, Rowland, & Cunningham, 1998). Our model includes multisystemic levels (represented by a series of concentric circles) including: the individual, the family, the extended family, "nonblood kin" and other close friends, church and community resources, and social service agencies and other outside systems (see Figure 1.1). The last-mentioned circle deserves particular emphasis here, because family practitioners often discover that the families they work with are dealing with many complex problems and are likely to be involved with an array of agencies and institutions. These include schools, day care centers, medical or health care providers, mental health agencies, child welfare or protective services, welfare programs, housing authorities, and/or the juvenile justice system. Each client has existing relationships with such agencies, institutions, and systems, many of which may be negative, and most if not all of which will have considerable impact on the therapeutic relationship and the outcome of therapy.

Researchers and clinical scholars (Aponte, 1976; Aponte, 1995; Boyd-Franklin, 1989; Bronfenbrenner, 1977; Henggeler & Borduin, 1990; Henggeler et al., 1998) have found the multisystems model to be a pragmatic approach to understanding complex ecosystems. It allows workers to intervene at multiple systemic levels. It is extremely helpful in work with urban poor families, who may simultaneously confront a staggering number of problems: poverty, unemployment, drug and alcohol abuse, teenage pregnancy, low educational attainment, poor health (including HIV/AIDS), crime, and homelessness, among others. The multisystems model is also particularly useful in work with African American, Latino, and other ethnic minority families and communities, because it recognizes the impact of the dual sociopolitical stressors of poverty and racism or prejudice (Boyd-Franklin, 1989, 1998).

THE MULTISYSTEMS MODEL

Multisystems

Level I	Individual
Level II	Subsystems
Level III	Family household
Level IV	Extended family
Level V	Nonblood kin and friends
Level VI	Church and community resources
Level VII	Social service agencies and other outside systems

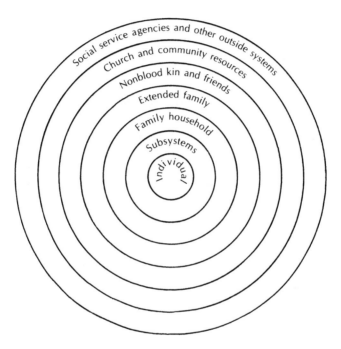

FIGURE 1.1. The multisystems model. From Boyd-Franklin (1989, p. 149). Copyright 1989 by Nancy Boyd-Franklin. Reprinted by permission.

REACHING OUT

Advantages of Reaching Out

The multisystems model is a useful theoretical framework for clinicians who do home- or office-based work because it allows them to conceptualize the realities of clients' lives in a more complete and complex way. By incorporating the process of "reaching out" (i.e., working outside the office), this model can allow the clinician to observe and intervene directly in the various systems that have an impact on clients' lives and that either support or hinder their progress toward achieving therapeutic change (Berg, 1994; Tatum, Moseley, Boyd-Franklin, & Herzog, 1995).

For example, a home-based family therapy session can give the clinician an opportunity to observe the client's and family's life *in vivo*. In office-based family therapy, we frequently work with only a subsystem of a complex family household and extended family network, not engaging with individuals who often have a great deal of power either to produce or to sabotage change (Haley, 1976; Minuchin, 1974). In home-based work, for example, we have the opportunity to engage and form a therapeutic alliance with fathers and boyfriends, who often do not come in for office-based sessions.

"Reaching out" also has a broader meaning. Too often a clinician or family therapist "joins" only with the family being treated. This may be a serious error, particularly when joining with and entering poor African American and Latino communities. Our stance encourages workers to go beyond a one-to-one relationship and actively intervene in the multiple settings that are significant in their clients' lives. Often a family therapist spends as much or more time talking to people *outside* of the family as talking to the client and family. This outreach may take place in a client's home, school, or day care center, or (if it is convenient or useful to the intervention) at a community facility or institution, such as a church, community center, or another common meeting place. For example, in order to meet an overburdened mother of preschool and infant children, a family therapist can arrange to be at the day care center during "dropoff time" in the morning. One can learn a great deal about the client and family's world through visits such as these. One clinician even went to the park where an adolescent regularly played basketball when he avoided meetings at home and school. This approach therefore allows the family therapist or worker to gain a more comprehensive view of family members' lives by "reaching out" to their environment and to significant others.

Reaching Out: Strategies for Clinicians in Office-Based Work

Many clinicians feel constrained by managed care plans that do not cover home- or community-based services, or by agency practice that focuses primarily on office-based sessions. The therapists in these situations can benefit from even one well-timed home-based family session and can increase the impact of ongoing office-based work. For example, if a key family member is resistant to coming into the office for treatment, this family member may be amenable to a home-based session, which can facilitate his or her "buy-in" (Henggeler et al., 1998) and support of the therapeutic work. Targeted reaching out can also be useful in major therapeutic efforts that require the participation of a large number of family and extended family members. For example, a drug or alcohol "intervention" (Treadway, 1989), in which key members of an individual's family, work, community, or church network come together to challenge the client's substance abuse and strongly encourage him or her to seek treatment, is often best held either in the home or in a neutral community center or church office (where all of the parties may feel more comfortable assembling).

Clinicians have often told us that they have saved hours of wasted "telephone tag" by paying a brief visit to a child's school during their lunch hour. Although a large caseload may prevent such visits on a regular basis, one carefully planned meeting may allow a clinician to connect with a principal, teacher, or counselor who has the power to make major decisions in a child's life.

KEY CONCEPTS

- The multisystems or *ecological approach to service delivery* (Aponte, 1995; Boyd-Franklin, 1989; Henggeler et al., 1998; Weissbourd & Kagan, 1989). The multisystems model allows us to view clients and families in their full ecological and systemic context, including the many different institutions, agencies, and systems that have an impact upon them.
- *Cultural sensitivity and competence* (McGoldrick, Giordano, & Pearce, 1996; McGoldrick, Pearce, & Giordano, 1982). Each intervention must be tailored to and sensitive to the cultural realities of the family.
- *Emphasis on strengths* (Boyd-Franklin, 1989). The emphasis is on identifying the strengths in the child or adolescent, parent, family, school, and community that can be utilized to produce change.
- *Empowerment of families* (Berg, 1994; Boyd-Franklin, 1989). This approach emphasizes supporting families in taking charge of their own lives. The clinician should not "take over" the job of the family.
- *Proactive and active interventions* (Bry, 1994). The role of the clinician in this model is a very active one. The therapist actively reaches out to family members and to systems, such as schools, child protective services, the juvenile justice system, the police,

and the courts. The therapist is proactive in the sense that he or she initiates contact and changes within systems, rather than accepting the situation and waiting for change to occur.

- *Value of support* (Schorr, 1997). Throughout this book, we emphasize the importance of support and support networks in the lives of children, adolescents, parents, and families.
- *Community involvement* (Boyd-Franklin, Morris, & Bry, 1997). The concept of "reaching out" in this book extends not only to families, but to the communities in which they live. Key community members and organizations can be involved in the process of change. For example, a church might provide a location for a family support group; a school might provide an after-school tutoring program; or a community center in a low-income housing project might provide general equivalency diploma (GED) courses or job training.
- *Prevention* (Bry, 1994, 1996). One of the most useful applications of the multisystems model and the process of "reaching out" involves interventions with children and adolescents who are at risk for the negative outcomes of conduct disorder, dropping out of school, drug or alcohol abuse, or gang activity or other trouble with the law. These can be prevented if targeted interventions begin at an early stage. Such interventions are described in Chapters 7 and 10.

CONFIDENTIALITY

We introduce the issue of confidentiality in this book because matters pertaining to ethics and confidentiality are particularly complex in multisystems family work and are of course integral to all interventions. The fundamental rules of confidentiality apply to all work with clients. Therapists should always be aware of professional guidelines and state laws regarding confidentiality, particularly when it pertains to information given by minors. Although family members should be comfortable in the knowledge that what occurs in therapy is confidential, it should also be made clear to them that therapist–client privilege is not absolute; for example, family therapists are required by law to report all cases of child abuse. Beyond these fundamentals, there are specific issues that need to be addressed in multisystemic family therapy. Three types of confidentiality are discussed in specific chapters: (1) within the family (i.e., between parents and adolescents) in Chapter 3; (2) between families and schools or other outside agencies in Chapter 7; and (3) between families and other individuals and families in their community in Chapter 8.

OVERVIEW OF THE BOOK

When we embarked on this project, our goal was to create a comprehensive resource that could be useful to both beginning and experienced family therapists in many different types of agencies and settings. This first section of the book presents the underlying values and principles of our approach. In Chapter 2, we discuss the importance of an understanding of cultural, racial, and socioeconomic issues for clinicians undertaking this work with families. This chapter focuses primarily on the cultural strengths of African American and Latino families, the two major ethnic minority groups with which we have worked, and on our interventions with poor families from many cultures.

Part II of the book focuses on home-based family treatment—an integral element of outreach. This section highlights work with families who are frequently "in crisis," and it describes interventions and effective parenting strategies with families of children at different developmental levels, including infants, preschoolers, school-age children, and adolescents.

Chapter 3 provides the reader with an overview of the guiding principles and challenges of home-based family therapy. Beginners will benefit from thorough discussions of the processes of joining, connecting, and contracting; the advantages of a home-based approach; and the importance of effective "use of self" in treatment. More experienced family workers will find useful the sections on working with challenges, especially "resistance," angry clients, and families with multiple problems.

Chapter 4 continues the focus on home-based work by addressing the needs of families in crisis. Case examples highlight multigenerational family patterns and the role of "toxic" secrets in such problems as teenage pregnancy, juvenile delinquency, and drug and alcohol use.

Chapters 5 and 6 encompass a developmental perspective on work with families of children ranging from infancy to adolescence. In Chapter 5, we focus on families with very young and school-age children. This chapter addresses issues such as child abuse and neglect, and discusses parenting practices and skills.

Our work with adolescents and their families is the focus of Chapter 6. A behavioral family therapy framework is described, and topics covered include understanding adolescents' behavioral motivation, the use of positive feedback, role modeling, monitoring, parental involvement, and advocacy.

Part III of the book addresses the need for outreach beyond the home—in schools, courts, churches, and communities. In particular, family workers must reach out to schools if they are to be effective in their interventions. Chapter 7 focuses on the ways in which family workers can approach schools and intervene more appropriately on behalf of their clients and families. This chapter includes a discussion of prevention work with high-risk adolescents.

Consistent with our emphasis on the multisystems model, Chapter 8 explores the need for family workers and other clinicians to connect effectively with the communities they serve. This includes the processes of joining and community entry. To be effective, family workers and their agencies must think beyond the individuals and families who are their clients and reach out to other key figures in the community. This chapter emphasizes creative ways to promote community development and empowerment; it focuses primarily on the use of parent and family support groups.

In order to explicate the concept of reaching out and the use of the multisystems model still further, a multisystemic case example has been included in Chapter 9. This provides readers with a more in-depth view of the overall approach.

The final two chapters, which make up Part IV of the book, emphasize the central role of research and evaluation in the development of effective services and the importance of effective supervision and training. Just as the multisystems model of treatment is an active one involving outreach, our model of supervision shares this emphasis on active, front-line supervision. We view training and supervision as "antidotes" to the burnout that so often occurs for front-line family workers, and as keys to the empowerment of clinicians to do this work effectively.

CHAPTER 2

Cultural, Racial, and Socioeconomic Issues

Client families are often faced with racism, discrimination, and poverty. In this chapter, we discuss the relevance of cultural, racial, and socioeconomic differences as they affect families in need of help. The primary focus is on the areas of our greatest expertise—work with African American, Latino, and poor families from White as well as ethnic minority backgrounds.

Practitioners are encouraged to view families and clients in terms of their strengths. Because clients and families in trouble present with their problems, understanding their cultural, racial, and socioeconomic realities can enable family therapists to search for and identify strengths in difficult situations.

Excellent clinical resources are available in the literature on many of these topics (Berg, 1994; Boyd-Franklin, 1989; McGoldrick et al., 1996). The goal of this chapter is to address crucial areas of intervention with these families that are often not addressed in existing publications. Although there has been a rapid increase in diverse immigrant groups in the United States in recent years (McGoldrick et al., 1996), we discuss only those with which we have had the most clinical experience.

POOR FAMILIES

Although socioeconomic issues are mentioned last in the title of this chapter, we begin our discussion here with a brief acknowledgment of these issues because so many of the families targeted by home-based family interventions and other forms of outreach are poor. Families living in poverty include a wide spectrum of cultural and racial groups, and reside in rural as well as urban settings. There has been a tendency in the treatment literature to equate families living in poverty with "ethnic minority" families. This is a serious error; there are also many poor White families struggling at subsistence levels in the United States.

Poverty should not be viewed as an independent variable. Readers are cautioned against adopting a "culture of poverty" approach that stereotypes all poor families. Race, culture, and socioeconomic level interact in complex ways that vary from family to family. Poverty is profoundly related to issues of homelessness, unemployment, lack of access to good jobs, high dropout rates, crime, dangerous streets, and communities with high levels of drug abuse and drug trafficking. These issues are exacerbated by the "double jeopardy" of racism and discrimination in the case of minority families. For some families, the interaction between poverty and racism may result in extremely negative consequences.

Poor families from all cultural and racial groups often perceive themselves as being at the mercy of the powerful systems with which they interact. This is true of many poor families, including those from ethnic minority groups. This can lead to frustration, anger, and possibly learned helplessness. Particularly for these families, it is essential that empowerment become a major treatment goal. To accomplish this, clinicians must avoid "doing for" the families, and instead empower them to take control of their own lives. This is often a gradual process. For example, for a parent living in poverty who perceives the school as a hostile, unresponsive place, the clinician can first role play interactions with the school in family sessions and then arrange to go with the client to the first meeting with school personnel. Ultimately the goal is for the parent and other family members to be able to make these school visits and interventions on their own.

Practitioners should be aware of the many "working poor" families of all ethnic and racial groups where family members have minimum wage or low-wage jobs with no health benefits. They may have large or extended families to support on incomes of $10,000–$15,000 a year. Serious illness, such as AIDS or cancer, can devastate such a family emotionally, physically, and financially. Important preventative medical interventions, such as prenatal and well-baby care, are often neglected. Some states now protect such families by providing Medicaid benefits for the children of the working poor.

AFRICAN AMERICAN CLIENTS AND FAMILIES

An important consequence of the experience of African American families with the history of racism and discrimination in the United States is the development of "healthy cultural suspicion" (Boyd-Franklin, 1989; Grier & Cobbs, 1968; Hines & Boyd-Franklin, 1996). This suspicion is often the first response encountered by clinicians working with these families, particularly in mandated home-based interventions. Multigenerational experiences with racism, rejection, and the intrusion of agencies perpetuated by the welfare system have helped to create in many African American families a view that family dynamics are "nobody's business but our own" (Boyd-Franklin, 1989). Members protect such families from intrusion by being secretive and sometimes unresponsive to outside interventions.

It is extremely important for a home-based family therapist, a school counselor or teacher, or a representative of a community agency to be aware of this perspective. Too often, an African American family is dismissed as "resistant," or a practitioner personalizes the family members' response and withdraws from them. The practitioner must be prepared for this and must be able to reframe it as an attempt by the family to protect its boundaries. It is crucial for the therapist not to take such a response personally or to feel that it is a commentary on his or her race, ethnicity, or ability.

A supervisor needs to be especially vigilant in helping a clinician to recognize that this initial response is merely the beginning of a chess game of engagement between the therapist and the African American family, and not a checkmate or the end of therapy. This realization is important both in cross-race and in same-race treatment. For White therapists working with Black clients, it is important to see "healthy cultural suspicion" as a factor to be overcome. African American therapists are often surprised when this suspicion also extends to them.

It is also important for clinicians to be cognizant of the cultural strengths of African Americans, which include the roles played by extended family members; the common practice of informal adoption; the desire for an education for their children, regardless of their feelings about the school system; love of their children and the desire to be good parents; and survival skills. All of these strengths are described in great detail in *Black Families in Therapy: A Multisystems Approach* (Boyd-Franklin, 1989), and therefore such descriptions are not repeated here, although the themes will be illustrated throughout this book in case examples. The following issues, which are essential for therapists to understand when working with African American families, are addressed in this chapter: (1) knowing who has the power in a family; (2) spirituality and religion; (3) expressions of anger; (4) parenting styles, including physical punishment and the issue of respect for parents or elders; (5) issues confronting young Black males and females; and (6) messages about violence.

Knowing Who Has the Power in a Family

When African American families are distrustful of outside agencies and systems, they may hide key family members from clinicians until trust is established. In addition, the concept of therapy is new to many African American families, who deem it appropriate only for "sick people, rich people, or White people" (Boyd-Franklin, 1989). As is universal across cultures, the most commonly presenting family group consists of a mother and one or more children. However, key roles are played in Black families by fathers and boyfriends, as well as extended family members (Gibbs, 1998; Gibbs & Huang, 1998) such as grandmothers, grandfathers, aunts, and uncles; therefore, an office-based therapist may not see the individuals in a family who have the real power to make changes. Well-meaning therapists can find themselves conducting endless family therapy sessions that do not produce change if those attending sessions are the least powerful members of their families. Paradoxically mothers and children are often in the least powerful family positions. When this occurs, therapists may be treating the wrong family members.

A home-based family therapist is thus in an advantageous position. By conducting sessions in a client's or family's home, such a therapist is more likely to encounter powerful family members in their own environment. It is very important to reach out to these individuals and to greet them, even if they initially pass through family sessions and go to another room. As trust develops, it is perfectly acceptable to say to a family member, "Perhaps your husband [father, boyfriend, mother, grandmother, grandfather, etc.] will feel more comfortable joining sessions as you get to know me better."

> For example, a team of therapists had been doing home-based family interventions with an African American blended family, in which the father and his son (age 15) had been living with his girlfriend and her two children (ages 12 and 13). Initially, when the therapists came to the home, the father would get up out of his chair in the living room and disappear into the back of the house for the entire session. (This was a metaphor for his role and behavior in the family.) After a careful discussion with their supervisor, the family therapists decided that they would take a proactive approach: They would greet the father at the beginning of the next session and invite him to stay whenever he was ready, because he was "so important to this family." He resisted for a number of sessions. Finally a crisis occurred when his son was suspended from school. Having laid the groundwork earlier, the family therapists were able to utilize the crisis to insist upon his involvement in helping them to help his son. This time he responded positively; he was greeted enthusiastically by the family and the therapists when he joined the session.

Spirituality and Religion

Different Meanings of Religion and Spirituality

Although the distinction between spirituality and religion in the lives of African Americans has been addressed in detail in a number of sources (Billingsley, 1968, 1992; Boyd-Franklin, 1989; Boyd-Franklin & Lockwood, 1999; Gibbs, 1998; Gibbs & Huang, 1998; Hines & Boyd-Franklin, 1996), many clinicians are still confused about how to utilize these strengths and resources in work with African American families. Certain individuals, particularly older female members, may be very involved in church attendance and have an active and supportive "church family." Others, usually males and adolescents of both genders, may be in rebellion against what they perceive as the excessively strict religious practices of some family members. Although resistant to religion as such, these same family members may have a "crisis spirituality," in which their early training or belief in God becomes activated when they are in trouble or in a crisis (Boyd-Franklin & Lockwood, 1999). Therefore, although religion and spirituality are tremendous strengths for many African Americans, it is important for the practitioner not to assume that they are present in all families or family members.

Differences about religion, spirituality, or their expression may cause intergenerational conflicts among African Americans. (See the multisystemic case example in Chapter 9.) When such a conflict peaks— for example, when a religious African American mother or grandmother is overwhelmed by problems caused by a rebellious child or grandchild—it is common for the religious family member to state, "I have turned him [or her] over to God." It is important for a therapist to assess whether this is a positive act of faith in which the parent or grandparent is praying for the child while continuing "parental" functions, or whether it represents a sense of giving up on the child.

Religion and spirituality have historically been essential components in the lives of African Americans. This can be traced to the tradition of African religions: "Religion permeated every aspect of the African's life. . . . Religion was such an integral part of man's existence that it and he were inseparable. Religion accompanied the individual from conception to long after death" (Nobles, 1980, p. 25). African American clients are likely to reveal their particular uses of spirituality and religion as coping mechanisms during the assessment process. Phrases such as "God will solve my problems," or "I am being punished for having sinned," are used commonly. Because of this intense spiritual connection, spiritual reframing may be a very useful technique in treating Black families. Examples of such spiritual reframing are as follows: "God will know what your needs are and will supply," and "He gives you no more than you can carry" (Mitchell & Lewter, 1986, p. 2).

There are many different denominations and distinct religious groups represented in Black communities within the United States, including Baptist, African Methodist Episcopal, AME Zion, Jehovah's Witnesses, the Church of God in Christ, Seventh-Day Adventists, Pentecostal churches, Apostolic churches, Presbyterians, Lutherans, Episcopalians, Roman Catholicism, the Nation of Islam, and numerous other Islamic sects. Of these groups, the Baptist and the African Methodist Episcopal groups account for the largest proportions of Black people. Even for African American clients who are not "religious," spirituality is such an important cultural value that it should not be overlooked in either the treatment or the community entry process.

The Role of the Black Church, Ministers, and the "Church Family"

Black churches have provided an escape for Black people from their painful experiences, serving as what Frazier (1963) described as "a refuge in a hostile . . . world" (p. 44). They were and often still are among the few places where Black men and women can feel that they are respected for their own talents and abilities (Billingsley, 1992; Boyd-Franklin, 1989; Boyd-Franklin & Lockwood, 1999). Black churches also serve a social function. Meals are often served on Sunday after services, providing an opportunity for families to mingle socially. Many Black single-parent mothers will tell therapists, "I raised my children in the church," or "He was brought up in the church." These mothers mean literally what they say: Black churches often function as surrogate families for isolated and overburdened single mothers. Many Black families, when moving to a new community, will quickly find a church as a method of becoming connected to the community. Ways in which some of these same strategies can be used by family therapists to help build new networks for isolated Black families are discussed in Chapter 8.

One of the most important "family" functions that a Black church serves is that of providing a large number of opportunities and role models for young people, both male and female. Black churches often provide non-church-related activities, such as Boy Scouts, basketball teams, youth groups, and so on. Because of the need for services in many Black communities and the deep concerns about the education of Black children, many churches have begun to provide day care centers and schools on the premises. These are community resources of which therapists should be aware.

In many parts of the United States, ministers have a great deal of influence both in their congregations and in their communities at large.

This is true in African American and Latino communities also. Among African Americans, for example, Black churches have historically been among the most viable institutions in their communities (Billingsley, 1968, 1992; Boyd-Franklin, 1989; Comer & Hamilton-Lee, 1982; Hines & Boyd-Franklin, 1982, 1996).

Ministers often serve multiple roles as spiritual leaders, counselors, community advocates, and political activists. For many Black families, the Black church functions essentially as another extended family—the "church family." The minister is usually a central figure in the life of a family and may be sought out for pastoral counseling in times of trouble, pain, or loss. After the nuclear and extended family, the church is the most common source of help among Black people.

A Black church may have a board of deacons and deaconesses who assist the pastor in carrying out the duties of the church. If a family member holds such a position in his or her church, this is clearly a strength and a sign of leadership ability. Black churches provide spiritual and social activities for the whole family. Sunday School and Bible Study classes are offered to congregants in all age ranges, from very young preschoolers to senior citizens.

Expressions of Anger in African American Families

In keeping with the "healthy cultural suspicion" (Boyd-Franklin, 1989; Grier & Cobbs, 1968) discussed earlier, many African American families present initially with anger directed at racism, at outside systems and agencies, and at practitioners. Although families of all races and cultures express anger in treatment, it is often more difficult for clinicians to deal with these issues with African Americans because of the dynamics of race and racism. An angry Black mother or father often elicits a fear response, particularly in cross-racial treatment. Although anger may be exaggerated as a test of whether the clinician can tolerate the parents' anger without withdrawing or abandoning them, another dynamic is that African Americans are often very expressive of emotions. Therapists from cultures that do not readily express emotions, particularly anger, may be frightened by this display. It is essential for therapists to be aware of their own response to anger and to seek advice from supervisors on understanding their clients' anger and not running away from it. (More information on how to deal with anger is provided in Chapter 3.)

Parenting Styles of African Americans

There is considerable variability of parenting styles within African American communities, based on socioeconomic level, parents' educational level, region of the country, religious practices, and generational differences. The parenting and disciplinary themes that are often difficult for therapists to address in working with African Americans may include "preaching," physical punishment, and the emphasis on "respect" for parents and elders (Boyd-Franklin, 1989; Hines & Boyd-Franklin, 1996).

Preaching

Desperate Black parents may resort to "preaching" to their children, unaware that children "tune them out." Compounding the problem, this preaching is sometimes accompanied by threats of extreme consequences that the parent expresses in anger but does not follow through with. This inconsistency between what is said and what is done is often problematic.

African American culture is a very verbal one, and clinicians may become frustrated with parents who cannot stop talking. The first challenge, particularly for young or inexperienced therapists, is to stop these parents from talking endlessly. Paradoxically, this can often be best accomplished by allowing such a parent some time to "vent" and complain in an individual session. The parent's venting of frustration and anger should be actively reframed by the therapist as expressions of the parent's love for their children and their desperation to find a way to help them. Messages such as "You have tried very hard," or "You really love him [or her] underneath all of your anger," are helpful in validating such a parent. It is helpful for therapists to affirm that parents have "tried to do the best they can" for their children, since parents often feel guilty about the problems of their children and are anticipating blame from therapists, schools, courts, police, and probation officers. Therapists may need the opportunity for feedback from supervisors, coworkers, or team members in order to find something positive in parents' actions.

Physical Punishment

One of the most difficult areas for clinicians, Black and White alike, in working with African American families relates to disciplinary practices that involve physical punishment, such as spanking. Often in response to the fear of negative consequences from society if children misbehave, many African American parents and grandparents have adopted a "spare the rod, spoil the child" approach to child rearing (Boyd-Franklin, 1989; Hines & Boyd-Franklin, 1996). A parent often says, "If I don't discipline him, the police will." Memories and stories of lynchings, beatings, and false imprisonment have been part of African American parental testimony for generations.

Clinicians are required under law to report incidents of child abuse. Therapists should not deny their responsibility to report child abuse when it occurs, nor should they collude with families to keep it a secret from child protective services. A more prudent position involves a careful questioning of the children and the parents about what actually occurred. A therapist must evaluate whether a "spanking" is within cultural norms or constitutes child abuse. Children or other family members may have exaggerated the degree of discipline by calling a "spanking" a "beating." Also, children, particularly adolescents, may manipulate parents by threatening to call child welfare or child protective services. Therapists from other cultures may want to seek help or consultation from African American coworkers in deciding whether the line of abuse has been crossed in such cases. These coworkers can then serve as "cultural consultants" for the therapist.

Clinicians treating families where discipline is problematic should acknowledge both the cultural parenting practices and the censure of child welfare laws. For example, a therapist may say, "Yes, I know that this is a cultural practice for you, but I'm concerned that if you continue to spank them, your children may be taken away from you. I care about you and your family, and I don't want to see you lose your children. Let's explore other ways of getting them to listen to you without resorting to hitting."

When a parent does need to be reported to child protective services, it is often helpful for a supervisor or administrator to adopt the "bad cop" position and state, "We have a legal obligation to report this." This allows the family therapist or worker to adopt a "good cop" position and support the family through the process.

Respect for Parents or Elders

Given the lack of respect with which they are treated in the rest of society, African Americans often insist that their children show respect for them. Sometimes "respect" may be defined so broadly by a parent as to preclude the expression of angry or upsetting feelings to the parent. Children's typical expressions of opposition (e.g., rolling their eyes, sucking their teeth, turning their backs, or cursing) can often be met with intense anger and physical retribution by some Black parents. A therapist may need to work with a parent or parental figure and the child individually before these issues can be addressed in a joint family session. The goal of the initial individual work is to create a climate in which the therapist joins with the parent(s) and the child or adolescent, validates each party, and empathizes with each. This process is a challenge that often taxes the therapist's conflict mediation skills. The therapist negotiates with the parent(s) to allow the child to express anger, on the grounds that it will not be allowed to fester and thus be acted out in school or in the community. Once a child has an individual alliance with the therapist, the child can be helped to see that he or she can express anger to the parents "respectfully" (i.e., without cursing, eye rolling, or "getting loud"). All of these issues are particularly intense when they involve Black male children.

It is also important for family therapists to remember that many African Americans are very sensitive about how we address them. This is particularly true of older family members. It is often best to start with "Mr." or "Miss" or "Mrs." or to ask "What name would you like me to call you?" before taking liberties with first names. In some of the case examples in the book, we have followed the family members' preference as to how they would like to be addressed.

Issues Confronting Young Black Males and Females

African Americans are especially concerned about the survival of their male children, given the punitive ways in which mainstream society reacts to Black males. This process can begin at a very early age. Black male children are disproportionately labeled when they are as young as 5 or 6 as "hyperactive," "aggressive," "distractible," "emotionally disturbed," "maladjusted," or "conduct-disordered," and placed in special education classes. Kunjufu (1985) describes a "fourth-grade failure syndrome," predicated on the fears of teachers and school officials. Unfortunately, in urban school systems, this process may occur as early as kindergarten or first grade.

Black parents are thus often extremely suspicious of the motives of school authorities, police, juvenile justice officials, courts, and probation officers. In an attempt to protect their children from acts of authorities that are perceived as racist, Black parents may adopt a "not my child" position even when their children are in the wrong.

Therapists are often surprised by and unprepared for this reaction in parents. Parents with multigenerational experiences of problems with a school system may automatically take an adversarial position in response to a call from their child's school. Some parents feel that the only way to defend their children is to "go ballistic" at school conferences. Unfortunately, this often worsens a family's relationship with the school, court, or police, and causes authorities to dismiss parental input or to adopt a self-fulfilling prophecy of "like parent, like child." A family therapist often has to intervene by joining first with the parent(s) and with the school separately before bringing them together. Once a strong bond with a parent has been established, as suggested above, the therapist can engage the parent in role play before parent–teacher conferences or Child Study Team meetings. For example, the therapist can say, "You want the school to take you seriously so that you can get what you want for your child. If you go in there and 'go ballistic,' they are going to dismiss you and take action against him [or her]. Let's rehearse how you can handle this teacher or principal and get the result you want for your son (or daughter)."

Many Black parents fear that they will lose their children—particularly their sons—to violence, drugs, incarceration, or early death. In their fear and panic, they often take extreme positions with their adolescents and with authority figures in their lives. Some families give up. For example, in a family session in the home, a therapist asked whether the parent was aware of her adolescent daughter's repeated suspensions. The parent responded that she was "fed up"; as the stunned therapist looked on, she went to a nearby drawer and pulled out 15 unopened letters from the school.

A therapist may encounter situations in which a parent and a child have a "rep" (i.e., a negative reputation) in the school. Work often has to be done first with school authorities to allow them to vent their frustrations before the therapist can persuade them to give the family "another chance" and schedule a meeting. The therapist must work very hard to reframe even small positive changes and outcomes and to emphasize the importance of the fact that the meeting is taking place.

African American parents are all too often correct in identifying situations in which their children are discriminated against. It is not helpful for family therapists to deny this and enter into a power struggle with these families. A "both–and" approach is indicated—one in which racism is acknowledged, *and* the parents' help is sought in teaching their children how to deal with racism when it occurs and not be defeated (or feel victimized) by it.

Gender roles are complicated in African American families because of the perceived vulnerability and "invisibility" (Franklin, 1993) of African American males in society. As discussed above, Black parents, particularly mothers, often focus a great deal of their anxiety and fears on their male children. There is a saying that Black mothers "raise their daughters, but love their sons." This does not imply that daughters are loved less, but it does indicate the sense of anxiety and helplessness that many Black families feel about their ability to protect their male children (Boyd-Franklin & Franklin, 1998). As a consequence, girls are frequently given the message "God bless the child who has her own" and raised with an understanding that, because of the invisibility of Black men in society and the job market, they may be required to take care of and raise their families alone (Boyd-Franklin & Franklin, 1998).

Older girls and boys are often expected to function responsibly as "parental children" (Minuchin, 1974) and caregivers for younger siblings. These adolescents have often been carrying adult responsibility since their childhoods and are consequently less likely to accept adult direction and limit setting in adolescence. Parents and grandparents often complain that "they think they are grown."

Messages about Violence

One of the dilemmas faced by African American parents, particularly in inner-city areas, is the risk of violence to their children. Black children were traditionally given the message by parents raised in the era of fistfights that they should not start fights, but should defend themselves and fight back if provoked. (See the case of Kevin in Chapter 7.) However, Black parents today are haunted by stories of adolescents who become involved in altercations and are killed with guns (Boyd-Franklin et al., 1997).

Given the risk of street violence, young male and female adolescents are tempted to join gangs, or at the very least to align themselves with groups of other youth, in exchange for protection. This trend is often denied by parents, school officials, and juvenile authorities alike. Unlike adolescents of other cultures, African American youth frequently experience a sense of their own mortality. This point was vividly conveyed in a group therapy session in which a group of African American adolescents (ages 12–14) were asked to participate in an "I have a dream" exercise and to project their future dreams and hopes for themselves. One of the most intelligent, articulate members responded that he was convinced that he would be killed before adulthood.

African American parents are especially conflicted about what messages to give their children with regard to their behavior if they are provoked in encounters with the police. African American adolescents, especially males, are often targeted by the police and stopped randomly when a crime has been committed. Many Black parents, of all socioeconomic and educational levels, feel the need to prepare their adolescents for the ways in which they should and should not behave if they are stopped by the police.

It is very important for clinicians to be sensitive to the reality-based fears of these families. Also, this might be an appropriate topic for a family session if an African American parent has not had a frank discussion with a child about how to deal with police and other authorities. The family therapist can empower the parent to teach the child how to respond, in a way that will avoid problems. Boyd-Franklin, Franklin, and Toussaint (in press) and Gardere (1999) offer helpful suggestions that family therapists and parents can use to prepare their children for encounters with the police.

LATINO CLIENTS AND FAMILIES

The terms "Latino" and "Hispanic" are American terms used to describe families from a wide range of countries, cultures, and sociopolitical histories (Bernal, 1982; Bernal & Shapiro, 1996; Falicov, 1982, 1996, 1998; Garcia & Zea, 1997; Garcia-Preto, 1996), including the following cultural groups: "Cubans, Chicanos, Mexicans, Puerto Ricans, Argentineans, Colombians, Dominicans, Brazilians, Guatemalans, Costa Ricans, Nicaraguans, Salvadorians, and all other nationalities that comprise South America, Central America, and the [Spanish-speaking] Caribbean" (Garcia-Preto, 1996, p. 142). Many of these individuals identify themselves by their place of origin—for example, "I am Puerto Rican," or "My family is from Cuba"—rather than as "Latino" or "Hispanic."

Although the countries collectively known as "Latin America" share Spanish as their common language (with the exception of Portuguese-speaking Brazil), many differences exist in terms of the idiomatic use of language, customs, and traditions (Falicov, 1996, 1998; Garcia-Preto, 1996). Latino families also include individual family members who are at different points along the immigration/acculturation continuum. Evelyn Lee (1996) has presented a schema of this acculturation continuum. Although her work has been with Asian Americans, it provides a very useful framework for viewing all clients and families who have immigrated to the United States. Her continuum of families in transition encompasses the following categories: "traditional" families, "cultural conflict" families, "bicultural" families, "Americanized" families, and "interracial" families.

For Latinos, this continuum requires modification to include the category of *undocumented* families, whose members include individuals residing in the United States illegally; such persons live with the constant fear of discovery and deportation (Falicov, 1996). Many have braved hazardous conditions in order to enter this country. Such "families" may comprise a communal unit of children and adults who may or may not be biologically related. It is not uncommon for 10–20 people to live together in a three-bedroom house or apartment. These families often live in an "underground community" and may have purchased false identification (e.g., a Social Security card, driver's license, or a "green card"), which allows them to live and work in the United States. Often these families come to the attention of authorities when their children enroll in school or when a family member becomes ill and is taken to a hospital.

Recent immigration laws (e.g., Proposition 187, an initiative passed in California in 1994) have been more punitive toward the population of undocumented residents, creating severe sanctions for these families (Falicov, 1996). Individuals who are not American citizens are not entitled to welfare benefits, Medicaid, or Medicare. Fear of deportation is a constant reality for these families, and any outsiders (including family therapists or family workers of any kind) may be perceived as a threat to such a family's survival.

For the purposes of this chapter, Latino *traditional families* (Garcia-Preto, 1996; Lee, 1996) consist entirely of family members born and raised in Spanish-speaking South and Central American and Caribbean countries. These family members still practice traditional customs and often speak primarily in Spanish (Lee, 1996). Much of the literature on Latino families has focused on this group whose cultural traditions and language are the most different from those of the American mainstream (Bernal & Gutierrez, 1988; Comas-Díaz & Griffith, 1988; Garcia-Preto, 1996). Traditional families often come for mental health and social service interventions via referrals from medical practitioners. A medical problem is often a much more accepted and comfortable way to express psychological or emotional pain or family problems.

Cultural conflict families either have American-born children or "arrived more than a decade ago when the children were young. The family system usually experiences a great deal of cultural conflict between the acculturated children and the traditional parents or grandparents" (Lee, 1996, p. 232; see also Inclan & Herron, 1998; Ramirez, 1998). If one spouse becomes acculturated more rapidly than the other, traditional gender role expectations may also be challenged (Garcia-Preto, 1996). This group is the one most frequently referred by schools and child welfare departments.

Bicultural families consist of well-acculturated parents who grew up in Latin American, Central American, or Caribbean cities or who were born in the United States but raised in traditional families (Comas-Díaz & Griffith, 1988; Garcia-Preto, 1996). These families are often of a middle- or upper-class background; the parents have professional jobs, and the families live in the suburbs. They are frequently bilingual and bicultural and have begun to modify traditional cultural expectations. Lee (1996) points out that many of these families have modified the patriarchal gender roles of traditional families and now have a more egalitarian parental relationship. Some of these families still have extended family members living in the household, whereas others have moved to a more nuclear family dwelling but still maintain frequent contact with extended family members.

Americanized families often consist of "parents and children born and raised in the United States" (Lee, 1996, p. 233). These families may also consist of different members at different points in the acculturation continuum. In some of these families, individual members do not retain their ethnic identities, and family members communicate largely in English. Many children, adolescents, and young adults in these families do not speak Spanish. These families are frequently upwardly mobile. Children often report being perceived as different from their high school peers, but they have no strong cultural identity with which to identify in order to reinforce their self-esteem and pride. Many of these youth act out this sense of loss in their adolescence. Sometimes young people in these families reconnect with their culture and language during their college years.

The last category, *interracial families* (Lee, 1996), might be more appropriately termed *cross-cultural* or *cross-racial* families because many Latinos are "interracial" in the strict sense of the word; some of their backgrounds may incorporate White European, African, and indigenous Indian races and cultures (Garcia-Preto, 1996). Cross-cultural or cross-racial families are those in which someone has married a person who is not of Latino origin. Some mixed marriages result in families in which children grow up experiencing the best of both cultures. Others struggle with conflicts in values, in religious beliefs, in language and child-rearing issues, and in expectations of extended family involvement.

Language Issues

There are many traditional and cultural conflict families in which all of the adults in the household (parents, grandparents, extended family members, and newly arrived friends or boarders) speak only Spanish. Often these older relatives live in "barrios" where everyone speaks Spanish. Their oldest child may be the only member of the household whose English is sufficient to interact with the outside world (Comas-Díaz & Griffith, 1988; Garcia-Preto, 1996).

Inevitably, children in traditional families become more acculturated than their parents and grandparents by virtue of their contact with other children in school (Inclan & Herron, 1998; Ramirez, 1998). Parents, who are used to being in charge in their homelands, find that they cannot adequately fulfill key aspects of their parental responsibilities. Because of their education and fluency in English, children are called upon by family members to shop; fill out forms and applications; handle banking; and serve as translators for their parents in stores, schools, hospitals, courts, and mental health centers. This reversal of generational roles may give older children or adolescents an excessive amount of responsibility at a young age and expose them prematurely to adult concerns (Comas-Díaz & Griffith, 1988; Garcia & Zea, 1997; Garcia-Preto, 1996; Gibbs & Huang, 1998). Having assumed adult roles from childhood, many of these adolescents become defiant when parents attempt to set limits and impose parental control. They may become resentful of family responsibilities in adolescence, feeling that they were deprived of the more carefree childhoods enjoyed by some of their American friends. These clashes of values can lead to other generational conflicts as well.

It is very important that English-speaking family therapists avoid using such parentified children as translators in family sessions. Agencies should be pushed to hire bilingual therapists. If this is not possible, parents can be encouraged to bring a trusted relative or friend to translate for them.

Generational Issues and Adolescent Conflicts

As the preceding section has indicated, differences in the level of acculturation can lead to generational conflicts between Latino parents and their children. At no time is this more pronounced than during adolescence (Garcia-Preto, 1996; Inclan & Herron, 1998; Ramirez, 1998). Part of the problem for these families, particularly those from an agrarian society, is that the life stage of "adolescence" did not exist in the same form in their homelands. Because of the expectations in their countries of origin that girls would marry young and that boys would begin contributing to the family income early in adolescence, families expect this level of responsibility and maturity from their children. Because of the cultural value of "respeto," traditional families are horrified when adolescents openly disrespect their parents. The typical North American and Western European concept of "adolescent rebellion" is very new for these families (Inclan & Herron, 1998).

In a desperate attempt to control their adolescents' behavior, some families resort to traditional punishments that leave them open to charges of child abuse. This drama is often enacted around a family's concerns that an adolescent daughter is "wild." In many traditional Latin countries, dating in the American sense is simply not allowed. Young women are heavily chaperoned in order to protect their virginity. Traditional Latino families in the United States often get into power struggles with adolescents who see their more acculturated Latino friends and those from other cultures dating (Inclan & Herron, 1998; Ramirez, 1998). This can become a major issue in high school, where dating is necessary to partake of established rituals, such as attending proms and other peer activities.

Parents, even those who are bicultural and more acculturated, may object to cross-cultural (particularly interracial) dating. This can be particularly problematic for adolescents living in communities with few Latino adolescents. More acculturated parents may also be faced with rebellious teens who resent their lack of cultural identification.

Religion, Spirituality, and Native Healers
in Latino Communities

In common with African American families, many Latinos have strong religious and spiritual beliefs. In the case of Latinos, this is due in part to the overwhelming influence of Roman Catholicism in much of Latin America (Bernal & Shapiro, 1996; Comas-Díaz & Griffith, 1988; Falicov, 1982, 1996, 1998; Garcia-Preto, 1996). In many Latino communities, Catholic churches are served by Latino or bilingual priests, incorporate Latin music, and are an integral part of community life. In these instances, the churches can serve as a support system for families, particularly for newly arriving immigrants. In communities where Latino families feel alienated from the local Catholic churches—often because services are conducted in English or they do not feel otherwise welcome—they are drawn to Evangelical churches.

Evangelical and charismatic sects have experienced a tremendous growth in popularity in Latin America. Recent immigrants to the United States are especially attracted to small storefront churches, particularly those of the Pentecostal sect. It is common for the ministers of these churches to be from the homeland of the congregants, to speak fluent Spanish, and to offer music alive with Latin rhythms. These churches often have a great deal in common with small neighborhood African American churches. Other members of the church are seen as *la familia de la iglesia* (the "church family"). Catholic priests and Pentecostal ministers alike are often beloved and respected in their communities and can be important resources for families and support or community entry points for community intervention (see Chapter 8).

After learning about the formal religious or church affiliations of Latino families, clinicians should be aware that many Latino families have other strong "spiritual" beliefs not necessarily connected to their formal religion. For example, some families from Puerto Rico and some from other Latino Caribbean nations often have a strong belief in *espiritismo*, which is a belief in the spirit world. *Espiritistas* or "spiritists" may be sought out by members of the community for help with death, dying, and other loss issues; physical illness; relationship issues;

and parenting (Comas-Díaz & Griffith, 1988; Garcia-Preto, 1996). *Espiritistas* are also sought for "faith healing" by those who believe that illness is caused by evil spirits.

Santeria, a blend of African Yoruba religion and Catholicism, is practiced by many Cubans and other Latinos in the United States (Bernal, 1982; Bernal & Shapiro, 1996). Historically, *Santeria* evolved when African slaves, forbidden to practice their own religious beliefs by their Catholic slave masters, gave the Yoruba gods the names of Catholic saints. In Cuba (Bernal, 1982; Bernal & Shapiro, 1996), this religion is known as *lucumi*, and it is called *macumba* in Brazil. Clinicians working with families who are coping with death and dying or serious illness should also be aware that natural herbs sold at local stores called *botanicas* are often utilized by Latino families because of their belief in their healing properties. For example, families that have immigrated from Mexico will often seek the help of a local *curandero* or herbal doctor to recommend remedies for healing illnesses.

For families who believe deeply in these practices, *espiritistas* and *santeros* (i.e., practitioners of *santeria*) are respected local healers. They can often serve as important resources when combined with family therapy (Bernal, 1982; Bernal & Shapiro, 1996; Comas-Díaz & Griffith, 1988).

Gender Issues

Family therapists, even Latino therapists, often struggle with the gender expectations in more traditional Latino families. Traditional male gender roles are encompassed by the term *machismo*, which is associated with "sexual prowess and power over women, expressed in romanticism and a jealous guarding of a fiancee or wife or in premarital or extramarital relationships" (Comas-Díaz & Griffith, 1988, p. 208). Family therapists with a very different concept of gender equality may become so appalled by this patriarchal system that they overlook the beneficial provider and protector aspects of the male role in these families.

Women are socialized in the tradition of *marianismo*, based on emulating the model of the Virgin Mary (Garcia-Preto, 1982, 1996). Women are expected to be self-sacrificing and to remain virgins until they are married (Inclan & Herron, 1998; Ramirez, 1998). The role of motherhood and bearing children, particularly sons, is valued. These gender dynamics may cause problems in traditional families because many Latina women are able to find employment before their husbands in this country. This reverses the traditional gender power balance, frequently leads to conflict, and, in extreme cases, can result in domestic violence (Garcia-Preto, 1996).

Traditional gender role expectations can also lead to cross-generational conflicts in some Latino families. Because of the high value placed on maintaining a girl's virginity, the practice has been to marry girls off at a young age, often to older men (particularly in more rural areas). This can cause problems in the United States because marriage is illegal for girls in their early teen years, and a nonmarital intimate relationship may be considered statutory rape according to some state laws. An especially problematic situation arises when a girl becomes pregnant in this country and is forced by the family to marry the baby's father. Some therapists may find it difficult to work with family members who make a pregnant daughter enter marriage in this way. It is important for therapists in this position to seek supervision from someone who understands traditional Latino cultural practices.

Another way in which traditional gender roles can clash with mainstream American expectations relates to education, particularly of teenage girls. A traditional or newly immigrated Latino family may encourage an adolescent daughter to drop out of school to take care of the home and younger siblings while both parents are working. In some traditional families, higher education is not seen as important for young women because of the expectation that they will marry and become mothers at an early age. This creates conflicts with school authorities.

Intense conflict can also occur when acculturated women marry traditional men (Garcia-Preto, 1996). A Latina who was born in this country, or who has spent the majority of her life in the United States, may have expectations of more egalitarian gender roles and the sharing of family chores, tasks, child rearing, and other responsibilities. These values may be in direct conflict with the more patriarchal expectations of her husband.

Family Difficulties Created by the Immigration Process

One common scenario for Latino immigrant families has been the experience of parents (often mothers) who leave children behind in the care of extended family members in their country of origin. Frequently, parents come (together or separately) to the United States on a travel visa or enter this country illegally. They must then find employment and someone who will sponsor them, usually an employer, for a "green card." The "green card" is a permit that allows an individual from another country to live and work in the United States. After obtaining a green card, a person can "sponsor" or bring other family members to the United States. Unfortunately, this process can take 6–7 years (or more). In addition, it may take another 6–7 years for the parent(s) to save enough money to bring over each of their children. Children left behind at a young age may well be teenagers by the time they are reunited with their parent(s). Other children may have been born here in the meantime and may have a closer or different relationship with the parent(s).

When family practitioners work with such a family in treatment, or school officials encounter such a family in school, it is common for them to be unaware initially of this complicated history. A parent may have had no experience in parenting and may be abruptly confronted with a rebellious adolescent whom he or she hardly knows. This is often exacerbated by an immigration requirement that a parent not leave the United States until the entire "green card" process is complete, which may entail a forced absence of 6–7 years during which the parent cannot return to the country of origin. This is particularly difficult for immigrant parents when their children are ill or when an older family member has died and they cannot attend the funeral. Many of these parents harbor a great deal of guilt about the length of time for which they are separated from their children and other family members. The following case example illustrates many of these points.

Case Example

The Martinez family consisted of Juan (age 16), Angelica (age 10), and their mother, Lourdes (age 32). The family was referred for treatment by Juan's probation officer after he ran away from home and broke into an office building in order to have a warm place to sleep. He was charged by the court with breaking and entering and was put on probation, with the strong threat of being sent to a juvenile detention facility if he violated his probation.

Family History. The family was from Nicaragua. Lourdes had become pregnant with Juan as an adolescent and given birth to him at age 16. Given the cultural belief in virginity until marriage (*marianismo*), her family was furious. They attempted to force Juan's father to marry Lourdes, but were unable to do so because he was already married. Her parents then sent her to live in New Jersey with a cousin while her parents raised her baby in Nicaragua. Through her cousin, who was in the United States illegally, Lourdes was able to find employment as a live-in babysitter with a family here, whose members later sponsored her for her "green card."

She told the family worker that these were very difficult years for her. Because of the "green card" process, she was unable to leave the country for many years in order to see Juan. Her father became very ill, and she was unable to visit him before he died or to attend his funeral.

Every payday, Lourdes sent money back to her mother in Nicaragua for the care of her child. She often sent barrels containing food and gifts, and always sent presents for Christmas and birthdays.

In the last year of her "green card" process, Lourdes met a man from Colombia with whom she became involved. They lived together on weekends, when she had time off from her live-in babysitting job. This man was abusive to her, and she soon found out that he was a drug dealer employed by a drug cartel. She ended her relationship with him after discovering that she was pregnant. Her second child, Angelica, was born just as she completed her "green card" process. Lourdes continued her live-in job and kept her child with her. She bonded closely with her baby but felt very lost without Juan.

When the child she was caring for as a live-in babysitter grew too old to need a full-time caretaker, her employer let her go. The family she subsequently found work with would not permit her to bring Angelica to live with her. When Lourdes flew home to Nicaragua to leave Angelica with her mother, she saw Juan for the first time in almost 9 years.

Because of Lourdes's hard work and frugality, within 4 years she was able to afford her own apartment and to bring her children to live with her. By this time, Juan was 13 and Angelica was 7. When they returned to the United States, Lourdes was quickly overwhelmed by the demands of working full-time and raising two children. She connected well with Angelica, with whom she had bonded for a number of years after her birth. However, her relationship with Juan was problematic from the start.

Whereas his sister was bright and cute, quickly made friends, and began learning English in school, Juan experienced many more adjustment difficulties. Whereas Angelica was close to her mother, Juan longed for his grandmother, Julia, whom he considered "Mama." He grieved for her loss, became increasingly depressed and angry, and withdrew from his mother and his sister.

Juan also experienced many difficulties in school. He had a great deal of trouble learning English in his junior high school. He had been in a rural school in Nicaragua and had never been exposed to the complex subjects he was required to take here. He began acting out and had behavior problems at home and in school. He failed his first year of school in this country and was forced to repeat his grade. This time, however, he was transferred to a school that had an English as a Second Language (ESL) program. He was befriended by his teacher and did much better that year.

His transition to high school was very difficult. He was sent to a large high school that did not have an ESL program. He missed his teacher and became more and more angry, acting out in school and at home. He became part of a "posse" of boys in school, and began to get involved in more and more fights.

By the time of the referral, the relationship between Juan and his mother was fraught with difficulty. He refused to accept discipline or limit setting from her, telling her that she was not his "real mother" and that she did not know him. Lourdes felt extremely guilty about having left him behind and totally overwhelmed by his behavior.

Treatment Process. The family therapist engaged both Lourdes and Juan. He found that he had to do this individually at first, because they were so alienated from each other. Gradually he was able to have a number of home-based family sessions that included Lourdes, Juan, and Angelica.

One weekend Juan "destroyed" the couch in the living room and broke a number of lamps after an angry argument with his mother. Soon after this, in a session, Juan angrily accused his mother of not loving him and only caring about Angelica. The therapist moved Juan and Lourdes as close together as they could tolerate and asked her to talk to him about this. She sobbed as she told him that she did love him very much, but that he seemed like a stranger whom she did not understand. He was able to tell her that she also seemed like a stranger to him. Lourdes was able to say that she wanted desperately to love him, to help him, and to be close to him. She told him that she felt very guilty about leaving him behind in Nicaragua.

The therapist asked Juan whether he had ever heard the story of why his mother left him with his grandparents. Both mother and son seemed surprised by this question and reported that they had never talked about it. With some help from the therapist, Lourdes was able to share with Juan that she had been very young when she had him (his current age of 16), and that her family had been embarrassed and furious with her when she became pregnant. She told him how she had been sent to live with her cousin in the United States. Both cried as she described how hard it had been for her to leave him and how she had cried every night for many years. Juan seemed surprised by this. They were able to hold each other for a brief moment as tears spilled down both of their faces. This session was a turning point in their relationship.

The therapist then worked closely with Lourdes on effective parenting skills. Up to now, she had felt so guilty that she had been inconsistent in her limit setting with Juan. She would tell him he was punished and had to stay in for a month, and then take him off punishment the next day. His probation officer, a White male, had taken a real interest in him, and Lourdes was encouraged to invite him to a session so that she could ask for his help in working with Juan. To her surprise, he offered to "take him out sometimes to play baseball" and eventually became a male role model for Juan.

Juan's relationship with his school remained problematic. He still had trouble with English and was failing many of his courses. The family therapist explained to his mother the process of requesting psychological testing and a Child Study Team evaluation. At first, Lourdes was overwhelmed at the prospect of going to meetings at his school. She had avoided answering letters requesting her participation because her English proficiency was limited and because she was overwhelmed by the size of the high school.

The family therapist asked her whether she had a friend or relative who could help translate for her. She responded that she had a friend who would come with her. The family therapist and this friend accompanied Lourdes to a meeting at the school. Lourdes was able to request the evaluation, and the therapist was able to emphasize that it would be helpful if Juan were given a Spanish version of the psychological tests and a bilingual examiner. He also requested that the school consider transferring Juan to a smaller alternative school that had an ESL program. After the testing was complete, the Child Study Team agreed to this request.

After this change, things began to improve for Juan. In the new school, he was placed in a smaller class, and the ESL teacher worked with him on his language skills. He was also away from the acting-out peer group that he had been drawn to. His behavior improved at home as Lourdes became more consistent in her parenting. His probation officer advocated for the end of his probation but continued to be involved with him, taking him to baseball games. The family therapist continued to check in once per month for a "booster" session for the first 2 months.

DISCUSSION

Clinicians are encouraged to use their knowledge of cultural, racial, and socioeconomic issues as a lens through which to view their clients and families. In order to avoid stereotyping, this lens must be adjusted for each new client and family. Clinicians must bear in mind that there is considerable diversity among poor families, and must carefully assess each family's needs and resources.

PART II

HOME-BASED THERAPY

CHAPTER 3

A Framework for Home-Based Family Treatment

Home-based family treatment offers a rare opportunity to observe family interactions *in vivo*, and it provides significant advantages over office-based family treatment. For example, office-based family therapists often struggle to engage key family members who are reluctant to come into an office. As shown in Chapter 2, reluctance to attend office treatment sessions is common among ethnic minority families, but it can be heightened in immigrant families (Falicov, 1996; Garcia-Preto, 1996). In particular, family members who are undocumented and are residing illegally in the United States are terrified of deportation and may therefore avoid social service agencies and institutions, such as hospitals and schools. Once a family therapist has established trust, these family members may feel safe enough to take part in sessions, particularly if they can be scheduled in the home.

As introduced in Chapter 1, there are six key areas in which home-based treatment may be preferable to office-based treatment (Berg, 1994). It provides the family worker with the opportunity to do the following:

- Meet important members of family, extended family, and friend support networks, most of whom would be unlikely to attend an office session.
- Engage the truly powerful figures in the family in the treatment process.
- Get a firsthand view of the family's living situation (especially of

such realities as poverty, substandard housing, drugs, overcrowding, crime, and an unsafe neighborhood).

- Be exposed to the culture of the family (i.e., food, music, language, support system, religion, spirituality, etc.).
- Observe the family's child-rearing practices.
- Experience the family's home through the members' eyes.

This chapter provides a framework for conducting home-based family therapy. Basic principles are presented, followed by suggestions for meeting the challenges of this approach. Next, the four stages of a home-based therapy session are discussed. The chapter concludes with a discussion of street awareness and personal safety for therapists doing home-based work.

GUIDING PRINCIPLES

The guiding principles for conducting home-based family interventions are as follows:

1. Remember your own "home training."
2. You are on the clients' "home turf."
3. When in doubt, join.
4. Never underestimate the power of praise.
5. The effective use of self is the most powerful technique.
6. Empowerment is the goal, not helping.

Each of these guiding principles is discussed below.

Remember Your Own "Home Training"

Family therapists can benefit greatly from the exercise of putting themselves in the family members' position and considering how they might feel if a stranger came into their home asking painful, difficult, and sometimes intrusive questions. Imagine further that the person is there without their invitation or permission but at the behest of an outside authority, such as the courts, and that they are mandated to comply. Given this complex context, it is not unusual for family members to be guarded and uncomfortable in the first home-based session. Family therapists can do a great deal to put family members at ease during this first contact. Never underestimate the value of a pleasant personality; personal warmth will help put family members at ease.

You Are on the Client's "Home Turf"

Unlike an office- or clinic-based family session in which the family comes into the therapist's environment, in a home-based session the therapist is entering the family's world (Berg, 1994; Tatum et al., 1995). For family therapists or workers, used to orderly home environments or structured sessions, home-based interventions can present a number of challenges. One rule for the first session is to learn to "go with the flow" of the family. Do not be in a hurry on a first visit to impose rules or your own sense of order. Try to relax, fit in, and get to know all of those present. An error sometimes made by beginning family therapists is to try to draw too rigid a boundary around the family in a first session. If visitors arrive during your session, greet them, but do not plunge into an exploration of personal family matters without asking the parents or parental figures whether they are comfortable talking now or whether they would prefer for you to return later. Take your cues from the parents or parental figure.

Even when the family members are expecting the therapist's visit, the therapist is likely to find them in the middle of a normal family activity. They may be eating; children may be watching television; adolescents may be listening to music or dancing; parents with small children may be changing a baby's diaper or feeding a child. One of our student family therapists was surprised to find a grandmother at the kitchen sink washing her hair. Another was told that the visit was limited to 15 minutes, because that was all the time left before the relaxer needed to be washed out of the family member's hair.

In some families, the tone may change dramatically if the father or father figure is home. This is particularly true for families who are receiving welfare benefits, and who may be afraid that the family therapist will jeopardize their financial support by reporting the presence of a man in the home.

When in Doubt, Join

Sometimes eager family therapists or workers make the mistake of "getting down to business" too quickly in the first session. This is not indicated in home-based treatment. You have entered the family's home. Therefore, the first session may be more beneficially utilized by chatting in a friendly manner with all family members and getting to know them. We often tell family therapists in home-based work that their main task in the first session is to be allowed to return for a second session. This is particularly important when there is a mandate to work within a very limited time frame. Joining is one of the most important interventions, particularly with ethnic minority families (Berg, 1994; Boyd-Franklin, 1989). For example, some Latino families need to feel a sense of *personalismo* (Garcia-Preto, 1996); that is, they need to feel very comfortable with a person first before business can be done. Such a family may invite the therapist to join them for a meal if they are eating, or prepare a special meal as a way to welcome the therapist. If food or a soft drink is offered, it is good manners to accept, especially in a first session. Although many of us were trained as therapists not to accept "gifts" from families, Latino families may feel very rejected by a refusal to accept food or a small token such as a handmade gift.

Young children will often offer an opportunity for joining and entry. If the therapist would not consider it too distracting, sitting down next to a child, playing with a toy, reaching out one's hand, speaking and engaging the child, or inviting the child to sit in the therapist's lap can be a way to "break the ice." It is important to observe the family members' interaction and to be active at engaging and speaking to all members (Berg, 1994).

Never Underestimate the Power of Praise

Parents who are not self-referred and whose children are having problems often feel as if they are failures. As mentioned above, parents frequently feel blamed by others, particularly if their children are getting into trouble (Berg, 1994). This may well be the case when they are getting direct messages to that effect from outside agencies. Both in early joining sessions and throughout treatment, it can be very beneficial to find something to praise in the behavior of parents as well as children. Positive feedback, such as "It sounds like you have tried everything you could think of to help him," can be very helpful.

Families in which there are multiple problems often have trouble recognizing small gains (Berg, 1994). In such a family, the family therapist will often be the "receptacle of the hope" or belief in the possibility of change. Praising family members for small gains is an essential part of this treatment approach. When a child's problems are the focus of treatment, be sure to praise the parent as well as the child.

> For example, a parent was complaining unrelentingly in a session about how far behind her daughter was in her homework assignments. Despite passing test grades, her daughter had failed most of her courses the previous marking period because she had not handed in her homework. After trying and failing to help the mother see the progress her daughter had made, the family worker

finally told her, "You know, I've noticed a change. Somehow you have encouraged Martha to do her homework every night this week. How did you do that?"

One rule to remember is that praise should be genuine and sincere (Berg, 1994).

> The case of a family in which therapy sessions were court-mandated and the family members did not want to come for treatment illustrates this point. The family therapist made the following statement to the father, who was particularly resistant to attending the family sessions: "Mr. Watson, I really admire you. You've been very honest with me about the fact that you didn't ask for this help and don't want it. I respect you a lot for coming today, even though you didn't want to, and for being here for your son."

Family therapists should not be surprised or concerned if some family members resist their attempts at praise or positive reframing. Continue to do it anyway. Persistence in this approach will often eventually lead to a softening of the parental stance or attitude.

Reframing or the use of positive connotation (Boyd-Franklin, 1989; Minuchin & Fishman, 1981) is another effective tool. For example, parents or parental figures who may be feeling very frustrated and saddened by a child's misbehavior may cry during a session. These tears may be reframed as "tears of love" or "tears of strength," since some parents can view tears as a sign of weakness:

> An African American grandmother, who was considered a "tower of strength" by her entire family, began to cry in a session as she described her fears that her grandson would "follow in his father's footsteps" and become involved with drugs. As she began to cry, it was clear to the therapist that she was mortified by this. The therapist therefore turned to her grandchild and asked, "How do you feel when you see your grandmother cry? Those are tears of strength and love that she's crying for you."

The Effective Use of Self Is the Most Powerful Technique

Aponte (1976, 1995) and Boyd-Franklin (1989) have emphasized that the effective "use of self" is the most powerful technique that family therapists can learn. Clearly, this is important in all forms of treatment, but it is essential in home-based family interventions. The effective use of self is based on a therapist's good understanding of herself or himself. The family therapist's own treatment can be very helpful in facilitating this process. In training, we acquaint family therapists with genograms (McGoldrick, Gerson, & Shellenberger, 1999; McGoldrick & Gerson, 1985), or family trees, and ask each therapist to construct his or her own family's genogram. This is an extremely helpful process as our family therapists experience for themselves the complexity of this tool. By familiarizing themselves with the multigenerational issues in their own families of origin, they can anticipate how their own sensitive areas may affect their work with families, as can be seen in the following case:

> Janet was a beginning family therapist, who was working with the Johnson family—a mother, father, and two children, ages 5 and 10—that had been referred because of the acting-out behavior of Patricia, the 10-year-old daughter. The father was very authoritarian and judgmental, and often yelled at his daughter in sessions.
>
> Janet acknowledged to her supervisor that she was very frightened of the father and could not stop him or interrupt his "blaming" of his daughter. The supervisor explored with Janet what the father's behavior was evoking in her. Janet revealed that Mr. Johnson reminded her of her own father, who was also authoritarian and abusive. Janet also reported that she was working on these issues in her own treatment.
>
> The supervisor was then able to help Janet to distinguish between Mr. Johnson and her own father. Through the technique of role-play sessions with her supervisor, Janet gradually learned to join effectively with the father in this family, and to help him to connect more effectively with his daughter. She learned to use herself as a bridge to help Mr. Johnson talk to his daughter and listen to her concerns.

Empowerment Is the Goal, Not Helping

Beginning family therapists, particularly when given referrals of families with many problems, often feel that they have to "fix" or "solve" these families' problems. Although this approach to addressing urgent problems may be an excellent joining technique in the initial treatment process, it should not constitute the only method by which the therapist engages with the family. It is very important to impart to family members the tools that will empower them to interact effectively with other systems and begin to find their own solutions. With this in mind, family therapists must learn to give the credit to family members for the changes they make, and not to take the credit for themselves (Berg, 1994; Minuchin, 1974). Helping, if it continues for too long, may create a dependency on the family therapist or worker that is not healthy or helpful for the family in the long run.

CHALLENGES IN HOME-BASED FAMILY THERAPY

The practice of home-based family therapy presents a number of challenges for family workers—some similar to those faced by all family clinicians, others unique to or exacerbated by the nature of home-based work. This section explores a number of these challenges, including "resistance," angry clients, family conflict, and "multiproblem" families. Many clients and families, particularly in public agencies, present with one or more of these issues.

"Resistance"

The word "resistance" has been placed in quotation marks because this issue must be viewed within the context of the nature of the referral. As discussed previously, many of the families described in this book are not self-referred, but have been sent by schools, social welfare agencies, or police authorities. Some, under the jurisdiction of the court, are mandated to participate. The responses to mandated or forced treatment are often anger, resentment, and "resistance." When the decision is made by another party or agency, treatment may be viewed by families as a further intrusion into their lives (Berg, 1994; de Shazer, 1982).

Not surprisingly, families whose members did not ask for help may not be receptive to the services offered. These families and their referral sources are likely to view the need for treatment quite differently. When families feel forced to participate, they may view family workers as part of that coercive process (Berg, 1994; Henggeler et al., 1998). This difficulty is compounded by the fact that many family workers have been trained to work with families whose members are self-referred and seek treatment for help with a particular problem.

It is important that family therapists be trained to expect initial "resistance" and anger on the part of some family members at being forced to participate in treatment, and that they be prepared to work harder to engage these family members in the treatment process. Thus, they can react more positively and will be less inclined to take such responses personally.

Persistence is vital for such family therapists. Family members manifest their "resistance" in a number of ways. They may not arrive for their first appointment. In a home-based setting, they may not be home, or they may be home but refuse to open the door. They may also absent themselves from participating in the session by engaging in other activities (cooking, watching television, talking on the telephone, tending to a baby, etc.). Often the ability to establish rapport with such a family requires the flexibility to follow the pace and direction of the family.

Such flexibility is a necessary part of training in home-based family treatment.

When families vent their anger at their sense of feeling "controlled" by others—a fairly common experience during a therapist's first encounter with them—it is important that clinicians accept and validate these feelings, and not feel obligated to defend the past actions of their own or other agencies. In fact, it is often helpful for workers to distance themselves from past interventions (Berg, 1994; Kagan & Schlossberg, 1989).

Angry Clients

Anger Directed at Family Therapists

Clinicians should be trained to respect their clients' anger and to understand its causes and legitimacy. Anger is not only related to being forced into treatment; as shown in Chapter 2, it may also be related to trust–mistrust issues. Clients who have worked with a series of workers from a multitude of agencies have often experienced loss, frustration, and disappointment. Anger forms a shield and serves a gatekeeping function to protect them from getting close to new workers, whom they fear will only disappoint or leave them (Berg, 1994; Boyd-Franklin, 1989).

Clients may also use anger as a test to see whether workers can accept their anger. This is especially relevant when working with African American families, as discussed in Chapter 2. Family therapists' training should include role playing related to the issue of anger. Clinicians may acknowledge clients' initial distrust by asking them to discuss their experience. It is legitimate for a family therapist to validate clients' feelings and say something like this: "You are very angry over the way you have been treated in the past."

Another important guideline for family therapists is to avoid getting into shouting matches with clients (Berg, 1994). It can be very helpful for a therapist to demonstrate an ability to tolerate a client's anger without responding angrily. If family therapists feel anger coming on and are afraid of expressing this anger or insulting clients—a very normal reaction to an angry confrontation—they should respectfully tell the clients that they will return at a later time. The therapists should then seek a supervisor, administrator, or more experienced family therapist in order to process the anger so that it does not interfere with the therapeutic relationship.

In circumstances where a worker is continually embroiled in angry confrontations with a particular client or family, it may be helpful to try a cotherapy relationship in which a team of family therapists treat the family together. It may be useful for the supervisor to accompany the worker to a home session. After personally experiencing the client or family, the supervisor will be in a better position to offer suggestions as to how the family worker might improve the relationship. When a family worker feels that a relationship is so poor that it is unlikely to be improved or repaired, it may be helpful to have a case conference where a number of staff members work together to generate creative therapeutic suggestions. Comments should be framed in the most positive way. Agency directors and supervisors need to develop a creative, supportive learning environment for family therapists and workers.

If these approaches have been tried and a relationship between a client and a worker still has not improved, the worker should be encouraged to discuss the possibility of transferring the case to another worker. Supervisors should take great care to ensure that no family therapist is given a disproportionate number of very difficult clients.

Anger Directed at Children and Adolescents

In addition to situations in which a client's or family's anger is directed at a therapist or agency, anger may even more commonly be manifested during a session as conflict between one or more family members. In particular, a mother or father, fearful of being blamed for being a "poor parent," may be very critical of a child or adolescent during a family session. The metamessage to the therapist is "I cannot be a bad parent; he is a bad kid." Parents who have tried everything may report giving up on a youth whom they describe as "no good."

Therapists often become very angry at parents who are highly critical of their children or who seem to be scapegoating or rejecting them in the session. A common mistake made by family practitioners is to become angry and judgmental of the parents and to side with or defend the children. The consequence of this is that therapists may withdraw from these parents, discontinue family sessions, and focus on individual treatment of the children or adolescents. This is unfortunate, because the essential relationship between the parents and children and the nature of their communication style are not being addressed. In truth, many clinicians are afraid of the expression of anger by parents.

It is important for supervisors to provide clinicians with a safe place in which they can address this anger so that they do not become judgmental and withdraw from or blame parents. It is helpful for clinicians to attempt to understand the parents' motivation for their anger. For many parents, particularly those living in inner-city areas, their anger is a manifestation of their fears for their children. These fears include a feeling of "losing their kids to the streets," gang violence, random violence, drug and alcohol involvement, crime, trouble with the law, teenage pregnancy, and/or early death. Their anger may also reflect their feelings of powerlessness to protect their children from the enduring nature of racism. (See Chapter 2 for further discussion of these issues.)

One possible strategy for clinicians in addressing this anger in parents is first to empathize with their anger and then to reframe it as fear for their children. Here is an example: "I hear your anger at him for getting himself into this mess, but I also hear your fear for him. Tell me about that." When clinicians fail to reframe the words of these angry parents and join with them, they are in danger of dismissing the parents' role by becoming "child rescuers" and ultimately losing these families from treatment. It is important that supervisors be vigilant about this potential outcome. This should be avoided whenever possible.

Another strategy is praise. The following case example illustrates the process whereby a family therapist's persistent use of empathy, praise, and reframing was successful in softening a mother's extremely critical approach.

Case Example. Arlene, a 29-year-old African American single parent and mother of Tareek (age 15) and Duquan (age 10), was referred for family treatment by the courts. Tareek had been arrested during a fight on the local basketball court. Frustrated and angry, Arlene made very negative statements about her son in the first session.

ARLENE: I am sick of him. He is just no good. You want him; you take him. He can't live in my house if he's going to continue to do this crap.

THERAPIST: You really are feeling frustrated in your attempts to change his behavior. Tell me about what you have tried.

ARLENE: I'm sick of trying. I've had it.

THERAPIST: I hear you. You love him, you care about him, but you're sick of beating your head against the wall.

ARLENE: That's right, I'm tired.

THERAPIST: Yes, you've tried hard for a long time, and now you're tired.

ARLENE: I can't do it all alone any more. Take him—tell the judge to get him out of my house before he messes up his little brother.

THERAPIST: You know, Arlene, you and Tareek are not in this all alone any more. You've sought help. Now you have me. You and I are partners in figuring out how to help Tareek.

ARLENE: Partners?

THERAPIST: Yes, we're in this process together now. You two are not alone. We can work together. Are you willing to work with me to help him through this?

ARLENE (*after a pause*): I'll try.

It is very important for a family therapist not to lose an adolescent in the process of talking to a parent. Adolescents in these situations also feel judged or blamed and may appear angry, oppositional, and/or defiant in the session. The therapist in this case therefore made it a point to join with Tareek.

THERAPIST: Tareek, I get the sense that this has been a really hard time for you and your mom.

TAREEK: Yeah.

THERAPIST: Can you tell me about it?

TAREEK: Huh?

THERAPIST: Tell me about what this last week has been like for you.

TAREEK: Hell.

THERAPIST: What do you mean?

TAREEK (*angrily*): It's been hell.

THERAPIST: So it's been real bad for you.

TAREEK: Yeah.

THERAPIST: I hear you. Can you describe it to me?

TAREEK: No.

THERAPIST: I understand. You don't want to talk about it right now.

TAREEK (*shrugging*): Yeah.

THERAPIST (*looking at Arlene and Tareek*): So the last week has been really rough for both of you. (*Both Arlene and Tareek nodded their heads.*)

Family therapists should not be offended by the monosyllabic, often angry tone of many adolescents. As we can see in this dialogue, the therapist did not try to talk Tareek out of his anger and frustration. He took whatever the adolescent told him, validated it, and moved forward. At the end, he generalized the frustration to both the parent and the child. This began the process of drawing them together.

Families with Multiple Problems

Families referred for home-based treatment often present with many problems. This is a reality that must be acknowledged. When a therapist is faced with a family experiencing multiple problems, it is a normal reaction for the therapist to become overwhelmed and begin to view the situation as "hopeless" (Kagan & Schlossberg, 1989). Whether consciously or unconsciously, the therapist may begin to label the family pejoratively as "multiproblem" and assume that its members cannot be empowered to change.

This cycle is very unfortunate. Even the most experienced workers may become overwhelmed by a family's problems and be tempted to "bring out the cavalry" (Berg, 1994, p. 198), pulling in many different agencies and services in an attempt to fix all of the problems. This can lead to a multisystemic nightmare in which many agencies, all trying to help the client or family, give different and often conflicting solutions.

Berg (1994, p. 199) offers a truly elegant blueprint for charting a therapeutic course with families who present with many problems:

1. *Do Not Panic*! . . . be calm.
2. Ask the client what is the most urgent problem that he [*sic*] wants to solve first. Follow his direction, not yours. Be sure the goal is *small*, realistically achievable and simple.
3. Ask yourself who is most bothered by the problem. Make sure it is not you; you do not want to be the "customer" for your own services.
4. Get a good picture of how the client's life would change when that one goal is achieved. . . .
5. Stay focused on solving that one problem first. Do not let the fact that the client is overwhelmed affect you. . . .
6. Find out in detail how the client made things better in the past. . . .
7. Be sure to compliment the client on even the smallest progress and achievements. Always give the client the credit for successes.
8. When one problem is solved, review with the client how he solved it. What did he do that worked?

The first step begins within the family therapist. By remaining calm and not becoming swept up in the family's panic, the therapist can help to keep the family focused on one goal at a time. The first problem to be addressed should be small, manageable, and "do-able." By highlighting and validating the family's efforts, the therapist can build upon even the smallest success. The importance of good supervision in this process cannot be overestimated; the supervisor, consultant, or peers can help an overwhelmed worker gain perspective on the problems and help the family to set priorities.

STAGES OF A HOME-BASED FAMILY SESSION

To achieve the best results with home-based treatment, workers need to acquaint themselves with the protocol involved in such interventions. Jay Haley (1976), in a classic chapter on the initial interview, provides family therapists with a blueprint that can be applied to all family sessions. He divides the session as follows:

1. Joining or social stage
2. Problem stage
3. Interaction stage
4. Task setting and ending

Joining or Social Stage

The initial communication sets the tone. As noted earlier, family therapists should remember their own "home training" and exercise good manners by calling first, introducing themselves, and asking the families' permission to visit. Surprise visits should be avoided. When a family does not have a telephone, a note such as the following may be mailed to the home:

> Hello, my name is _____. I am a worker with [Name of Agency] and I would like to make a time to come and visit your family. I have time available on Tuesday evening at 5:00 P.M., June 14. Would this time be convenient for you? If not, please call me at _____ and I will be happy to schedule another time.
>
> If I don't hear from you, I will see you on Tuesday at 5:00. I am looking forward to meeting you.
>
> [Sign Your Name]
> (Boyd-Franklin, 1989).

If the arrangement has not been made by phone, however, it may take more than one visit to gain entry to the home. For example, difficulties with literacy (because of either an incomplete education or limited fluency in English) may preclude the family from reading the letter. Even if a letter has been sent and read by a key family member or parent, other family members may not have consented to the visit.

When a therapist is visiting a family, a certain protocol is indicated. First, the therapist should introduce himself or herself at the door, ask for the parent or family member who was originally contacted by telephone or letter, provide a reintroduction if necessary, and remind this person of the phone call or letter. It should never be assumed that an open door is an invitation to come in. The therapist might ask, "May I come in for a short while to meet you and your family?" or "Is this a good time for a brief visit?" (Berg, 1994).

It is helpful to allow the client(s) to take the lead and decide where the meeting should take place. A therapist should not follow children into a home without a direct invitation from a parent or parental figure. Each person should be greeted upon entry. Some beginning family therapists are so focused on the person(s) they came to interview that they forget good manners and do not address other family members or visitors in the home directly. Saying, "Hi, how are you doing?" is often a way of acknowledging each person in the home or family. The therapist should always include children and elderly family members in the greetings. A simple "Hi, my name is _____," or "Hi, I'm (give your name) and you are . . . ?" can be helpful to put family members at their ease.

The first session should not include a great deal of note taking. This is the opportunity to try to get to know all family members and visitors, and to establish trust.

Problem Stage

In the problem stage (Haley, 1976), the therapist identifies and assesses the issue(s) with which the family needs help. With a family whose members are not self-referred, it is often beneficial to articulate the reason for their referral in a positive manner, such as the following: "Mrs. _____, the counselor at the school felt that Johnny could do better in school. Many other children and families have been helped by our program, and she recommended that I talk to you about it." Family workers should be cautious, however, about aligning themselves too closely with the referral agency, particularly if a family has an adversarial relationship with that agency. If this is the case, family workers might want to make it clear that they are not from the referral agency—for example, by saying, "I know that you were referred by your child welfare worker [or other agency], but I am not from that agency and I'm more interested in how you see the problem."

In the problem stage, it is important to get the opinion of all of those present about the problem. Frequently a parent, often the mother, has become the "expert" on the problem and the family spokesperson about it (Haley, 1976). This person can take over the session and not allow other family members to speak. The therapist may intervene and say, "Thank you. That was very helpful. You've given me a good idea of the problem. I'd like to go around the room now and hear everyone's opinion about this." The family therapist can then ask family members individually to describe their view of the problem. This should include the "identified patient," but should not begin with him or her. If family members interrupt, the therapist might initially not intervene in order to observe this process, but if the interruptions persist, the family therapist can say, "You have many good ideas, but I need to hear everyone's opinion. Please hold the thought, and I will come back to you a little later."

Interaction Stage

The interaction stage is a unique aspect of the structural family therapy approach (Boyd-Franklin, 1989; Haley, 1976; Minuchin, 1974) that can be particularly useful in home-based interventions. Family members will typically talk to a therapist but not to each other. It is a very powerful intervention to ask two family members to talk to each other. A family therapist might say this to a parent, for example:

THERAPIST: Would you ask Johnny how he feels about school?

PARENT: Well, you heard him . . . how do you feel?

JOHNNY: I hate it.

PARENT (*to therapist*): See, I told you so.

THERAPIST (*to parent*): Can you ask Johnny to give us some examples of exactly what he hates about school?

PARENT: So exactly what do you hate?

JOHNNY: I hate the teachers. They pick on me.

PARENT: What do you mean?

JOHNNY: They accuse me of doing things I didn't do.

PARENT: Such as . . .

JOHNNY: Fighting, getting out of my seat in class. You know . . .

The family therapist thus becomes a facilitator, helping family members learn to communicate with each other.

Task Setting and Ending

In order to draw families into the treatment process, it is often helpful to assign a task at the end of each session that the family can work on in the interim before the next meeting (Haley, 1976). This is particularly important if there are long periods between sessions. A task should be straightforward and directed toward the family's empowerment. For example, the family therapist might ask a parent to visit the school once with the child and speak to the guidance counselor about the child's school performance. The parent should be encouraged to take the initiative in this area. Only if a parent is unable (or, in some cases, too frightened) to do this independently should the family worker offer to accompany the parent.

For a child who presents a behavior problem in preschool, the parent might be asked to spend a morning observing in the classroom, to talk to the teacher, and then to share the results with the family worker.

Sometimes the task is a "family task." As suggested in Chapter 2, the therapist might ask a Latino or Asian family, with members who do not speak English, to talk together and choose an extended family member or close friend to invite to translate for them in the next session.

Sometimes "family time" can be prescribed. This often works well before bedtime when a parent might be asked to call together all of his or her children and just ask them in turn to share how their day has been. Tasks such as this can help to facilitate family bonding and togetherness.

It is very important that the family worker follow up on these tasks at some point in the next session. At the end of a session, it is often helpful to summarize for the family members what has occurred and to help move them toward their positive goals, as in this example: "All of you have worked very hard today so that I could understand the things you have tried to change Johnny's behavior. We will work together to develop new ways in which the family can help him."

CONFIDENTIALITY ISSUES
IN HOME-BASED FAMILY THERAPY

Early family therapists recommended seeing the entire family together (Haley, 1976; Minuchin, 1974). This served to control confidentiality conflicts, because no private alliances were made between the therapist and specific family members. In our work with adolescents, by contrast, it has often been necessary to work with subsystems in the family (e.g., parents, the adolescent, the sibling group). We often divide sessions into three parts: seeing the adolescent (and sometimes siblings) alone, seeing the parents alone, and then bringing the entire family together. We also schedule individual sessions with adolescents, which are particularly helpful with those who are resistant to treatment. In these cases, the adolescent(s) and parents may be seen alone initially and coached by the therapist to communicate more effectively with each other. This can help to create a task orientation and problem-solving focus. They may then be brought together for a successful family session.

As noted by Robin and Foster (1989), "In seeing family members alone . . . the therapist risks suspicions about 'secret information' and alliances, which may damage rapport with the parents or the adolescent. Confidentiality problems may arise as well, as when a teenager confides major drug use about which the parents are unaware" (p. 45).

All family members should be explicitly informed of the therapist's stance regarding confidentiality, right at the beginning of the therapy. Our approach to confidentiality recognizes that a therapist, particularly when working with a very enmeshed family, may wish to help establish a boundary of some privacy for a child or adolescent. Bry and Greene (1988–1989) state that "therapists often wish to have the option of keeping some things that [an] adolescent tells [them] confidential" (p. 21). Clearly, however, a therapist must disclose information if children or adolescents plan to harm themselves or others. It is our practice to inform the whole family of these policies at the same time, so that the parents and the child(ren) hear the contract together. For example, we may say to the parents in front of their children, "I would like it if you would agree that I might keep confidential what your child will tell me. Of course, I promise to let you know right away if I'm concerned about harm coming to your child or to others" (Bry & Greene, 1988–1989, p. 21). We may add that sometimes there will be important information that the parents need to know, but the adolescent is not yet comfortable raising with them. In such a case, we offer the adolescent a choice between bringing up the issue with the parents (with the therapist's help) or having us raise the issue in a family session.

Our approach is consistent with one approach taken by Robin and Foster (1989): ". . . family members are told that information will be shared at the therapist's discretion, but that the therapist will respect members' wishes about what should not be disclosed unless this secrecy interferes with progress, and will discuss sharing of sensitive information with them in advance" (p. 46). Before a sensitive issue is raised in a family session, however, a therapist should work with an adolescent to ease the process. This may be accomplished through role playing, writing out the agenda for the family session, coaching, and working out a series of "signals" that the adolescent can give the therapist during the family session. We have found that direct signals, such as "I need your help to explain this," work well.

We have found that parents are generally very willing to accept these parameters. Although they may express curiosity about what happens in individual sessions with their children, they are usually relieved to know that their children are speaking frankly to a responsible adult, given the frequent breakdown in communications at home.

STREET AWARENESS AND PERSONAL SAFETY

One of the most sensitive issues in home-based family therapy is concern about personal safety. This concern, more than any other, has prevented some agencies from making home-based work available to clients or from establishing effective procedures for using this form of work with families. We feel that this very sensitive subject of personal safety must be addressed directly.

What are the fears in discussing this matter openly? First, mental health professionals are often concerned about offending families by articulating these concerns. Second, it is difficult for an agency to provide guarantees about safety, despite the often unspoken but prevalent worries of administrators and staff. However, to embrace home-based work as part of essential services, the same problem-solving approach must be taken to allaying fears and enabling therapists to do this work as to resolving any other dilemma. For example, many other workers and volunteers in other community-based agencies manage the same concerns that family therapists may have about personal safety. It is important for agency administrators to contact such agencies and organizations and to discuss how they handle the issue of safety. This is one way of developing an understanding of this issue for the community being served. There may be professionals and other persons in these agencies quite skilled in home-based interventions, who, if specifically asked, might be willing and able to do an in-service training session for family therapists. This would be a step toward managing the fear and safety concerns of home-based work. We are not saying that such concerns would be eliminated, but that they would become more manageable.

It is also important that agencies interview, recruit, and hire workers who are familiar with and comfortable in the communities they are to serve. In ethnic minority communities, this means a special effort to search for workers who reflect the ethnic, racial, and cultural backgrounds of these communities. In interviewing workers from other ethnic groups, it is very important to assess their experience with and comfort in doing home-based work in these communities. For student(s) or therapists who are new to this work, it is important to request placement at agencies with a reputation for good support and training in this area. With such training and support, family practitioners from all ethnic backgrounds can do very effective work and be attentive to their personal safety.

Preparing and Training Family Practitioners for Safe Home-Based Work

It is very important that family practitioners who do home-based work feel comfortable in the communities in which they work. Supervisors and trainers should be careful to ease the fears of new family workers. An emphasis on safety should be a part of any orientation session for new workers. Each agency should draft safety guidelines appropriate for the area. It is a good idea to provide new workers with a walking or driving tour of the community, so that they can see the basic institutions (schools, churches, community centers, etc.) that play important roles in the lives of clients.

One particularly effective way to train new workers is to have them accompany an experienced therapist on a number of home visits for at least a week or more before they are given their own caseloads. Many agencies, burdened by large caseloads, often omit this step. It has been our experience that such support for new workers is a very worthy investment. It is also helpful to have an experienced worker join a new worker on the first few home visits the new worker makes for his or her own cases, and accompany a new worker who may have safety concerns or other hesitations when an emergency home visit is necessary. Another safety measure that some agencies have taken is to employ a male driver for the agency car or van. He will then be able both to escort female workers on home visits about which they have safety concerns, and to transport families to the agency or to other locations for community-based support groups.

Practitioners must remember that many of the families with whom they work are very sensitive to the "vibes" they convey (Boyd-Franklin, 1989) and can sense fears and discomfort. Some clients may be offended if they feel clinicians are overly fearful about entering their communities. It is therefore very important for workers to help and support each other in gaining this skill and competence. In our program, we have found it helpful to use cotherapy teams, particularly for new therapists. This investment has increased self-confidence and skill in our workers and has helped to increase the effectiveness of our interventions. As each individual grows in experience, he or she can then assume a full caseload.

Safety Guidelines

The suggestions below are intended to serve as guidelines; they can, of course, be adjusted to suit each individual situation. These guidelines were prepared for our program by a psychologist-in-training who is also a former police officer.*

Prior to the Visit

It is best to schedule home visits during daylight hours. If this is not possible, make a trip to the area in the daytime to familiarize yourself with the route to and from your client's residence. Many agencies provide small, portable cell phones for their workers as an essential component

---

*We are very grateful to Ms. Donna Ricca for her help in the preparation of these safety guidelines. Donna's dual training, as a psychologist and a police officer, has been very helpful to our program.

of home-based work. If your agency does not, discuss this possibility with your supervisor. If this discussion is unavailing, you might want to purchase a cell phone yourself as an investment in your safety. Carry it with you at all times. When in doubt, call for help.

On the day of the visit, remind your contact person within the family that you will be visiting, so that he or she will be expecting you. (You might also want to keep a colleague, friend, or family member informed of your home visit schedule.) Be sure to get careful directions to the family's home. Try to blend into the neighborhood you will be visiting as much as possible. Wear casual, but respectful, clothing and comfortable shoes (try to avoid jeans and sneakers); stay away from wearing flashy jewelry or carrying valuable-looking items. It is advisable not to drive a new or expensive car.

Ask a Coworker to Accompany You. As stated above, if you are new on the job or you are visiting a family for the first time, ask a coworker to accompany you for the first visit or raise the issue with your supervisor. Ask other family workers in your agency for their guidelines and tips. If you take public transportation, try out the route in advance and be sure that you are aware of the train or bus schedule.

Arrival at the Client's Residence

It is helpful to look around the area before you park your car and again before you get out of your car. If possible, park in a well-lit, populated area. As you leave your vehicle and walk to the family's home, appear confident that you know where you are going (even if you do not). Do not carry so many items with you that you do not have one hand free. This will allow you to use your cell phone easily, if needed.

Safety During the Home Visit

Home-based family practitioners may occasionally find themselves in difficult situations during visits to clients' homes. The basic rule of thumb is that your safety comes first. Certainly, if your client or a family member becomes violent, excuse yourself and leave. You can always call the police for help once you reach your car. You can do little to protect other family members by remaining in a dangerous situation.

After the Visit

If it is dark when you are preparing to leave and you are uncomfortable, ask one of the family members to accompany you to your car. As you leave the residence, have your car keys in hand. Once you are inside your car, lock all doors and keep the windows rolled up. Place your personal items (purse, briefcase, etc.) on the floor and out of sight.

Helping to Train New Workers

As you grow in understanding and confidence, be sure to "give something back" by helping to train new workers at your agency. Invite them to accompany you on a home visit in order to learn from your experience. Share the stories of your own fears when you first started, and emphasize the increased confidence and competence you have gained in doing this work.

DISCUSSION

Although it may be disorienting or difficult at first for family workers who have been trained to conduct treatment "on their own turf" to surrender that degree of control and treat clients and families in their own homes, workers who make this extra effort will be amply rewarded when this intervention empowers clients and families to change.

CHAPTER 4

Multigenerational Patterns in Families in Crisis

Families referred for home-based family treatment often, as a common feature, function in "crisis mode." Because they present with so many serious problems (e.g., homelessness; medical crises; sexual abuse, physical abuse, and/or neglect; suicide attempts; and arrest or incarceration), such families often prove daunting for even the most experienced workers.

Kagan and Schlossberg (1989), who focus on such families in their book *Families in Perpetual Crisis*, point out that many of these crises are repetitive and multigenerational. Despite the array of services offered to these families through schools, government agencies, social welfare departments, and the like, the families seem to change very little over time. Concerned about this pattern, the authors have explored the function such continual crises serve and have reached the conclusion that they are sometimes a diversion:

> Living in a crisis oriented family is like riding a roller coaster 24 hours/ day; terrifying, energizing and addicting. Families in crisis manage to flirt with disaster and avoid feelings of emptiness and despair. If you have grown up feeling cold, worthless, powerless, depressed, crises make you feel alive. . . . With the threat of collapse or dissolution of your family hovering over you, any diversion, however dangerous, provides some relief. (Kagan & Schlossberg, 1989, pp. 2–3)

Another function of a crisis, and often also of the "identified patient" in a family, is to get help for the family (Minuchin, 1974). Crises can serve to bring in others, such as school personnel, welfare workers, or those affiliated with the police department or courts, to offer relief from the family's feelings of powerlessness. Kagan and Schlossberg (1989) posit that the behavior that brings interventions of others into the family members' lives may bring a measure of relief once others take control.

MULTIGENERATIONAL CRISES AND "TOXIC SECRETS"

Crises brought on by such events as death, serious illness, hospitalization, loss of a job, or divorce cannot be avoided even in the most functional of families. What distinguishes these normative occurrences from those in the lives of crisis-oriented families is, first and foremost, the repetitive nature of the latter. For example, any family experiencing a crisis may feel acute grief; families that operate in continual crisis mode, however, have become inured to loss and block the further pain. As Kagan and Schlossberg (1989) state, "Crises become a way of life. The roller coaster has started and there is no getting off. It is exciting and dangerous but paradoxically comforting" (p. 3), because it is familiar.

Thus, crises become a way in which some families learn to deal with painful experiences, memories, and past traumas. This has particular significance when coupled with the concept of the "anniversary reaction" (Pollack, 1970). For some clients and families, a particularly painful event, loss, or trauma that is left unresolved can trigger a reaction (often an unconscious one) as the time of year or anniversary of the occurrence approaches. These traumatic memories can then lead to repetitive acting out in an attempt to master the pain of the earlier experience or to avoid it. Many family members report being "in crisis" or feeling "out of control" during these periods.

Four common multigenerational crises are addressed in this chapter: (1) teenage pregnancy, (2) child sexual abuse, (3) juvenile delinquency and criminal behavior, and (4) alcohol or drug abuse. All of these issues may become "toxic secrets" (Boyd-Franklin, 1989; Imber-Black, 1993) that fuel family crises. This link between toxic secrets is a pattern whereby one or more generations may attempt to avoid the pain of an earlier trauma by keeping it a secret. Paradoxically, secrets are often "known," albeit on an unconscious level in some families. As a result, a child's acting out may be a repetition of a trauma suffered by a parent that has never been openly discussed. Ironically, the action most feared by a family—open discussion of such a secret—is often what leads to a decrease in repetitive crises.

TEENAGE PREGNANCY:
A MULTIGENERATIONAL PATTERN

Adolescent pregnancy may be a multigenerational pattern in some families, particularly in inner-city areas. There may be a family history, going back to a great-grandmother, of a young woman becoming pregnant at about the age of 15. As the adolescent girl in the present generation approaches that age, the family members often feel intense anxiety. If this is not discussed, addressed, and resolved, it can be "acted out" both by the family and by the adolescent (Tatum et al., 1995).

If a mother and a grandmother both became pregnant in their early teenage years, they often become hypervigilant and anxious as their daughter/granddaughter approaches this stage. Family members act out this anxiety in one of two ways: (1) They become overly strict, restrictive, and punitive toward the adolescent at the onset of puberty in order to prevent pregnancy; or (2) they seem to give up control of the adolescent girl, treat her as if she is "grown," and wait for the inevitable. Unfortunately, either of these scenarios can set in motion a self-fulfilling prophecy in which still another generation is caught in the trap of early pregnancy and parenting.

Therapists aware of this multigenerational transmission process (Bowen, 1978) can work to make it explicit. Through the use of a genogram, they can explore the intergenerational repetitions. The following case example* illustrates these points.

Case Example

Sharon Smith, a 17-year-old African American adolescent, was referred for family therapy during her last trimester of pregnancy. At the time of referral, Sharon was living with her maternal grandparents, Robert and Margaret Smith, and other extended family members in an inner-city apartment. Prior to her pregnancy and for the first 5 months of her pregnancy, she had lived with her mother, Susan; Susan's boyfriend, Ray; and her half-sister, Dawn, in a nearby suburb. Conflict between Sharon and her mother had become so intense that she had moved to her grandmother's apartment, as she had at various other difficult times in her life. The grandfather was severely disabled and uninvolved with Sharon's care and with the subsequent therapy. The grandmother was a powerful figure who dominated the lives of many generations of her family.

---

*Sections of this case are adapted from Tatum, Moseley, Boyd-Franklin, and Herzog (1995). Copyright 1995 by Zero to Three. Adapted by permission.

Although Sharon was enrolled in an alternative educational program, her attendance had been inconsistent, due to her unstable living situation and to medical issues related to her pregnancy. This pregnancy was Sharon's third. At age 14 she had had an elective abortion, and at 16 she had miscarried at 6 months' gestation. Her current pregnancy was considered high-risk because of her health history and toxemia. The father of Sharon's baby, Chris, was still involved with Sharon, although he was disliked by both her mother and her grandmother and was consistently discouraged from seeing Sharon or from being involved with his child.

The intergenerational themes regarding adolescent parenting and role confusion were immediately evident in this family. Sharon's mother had also been an adolescent parent; Susan had given birth to Sharon at 16. She had wanted to terminate her pregnancy with Sharon, but her own mother had discouraged her from doing so and had been very involved in Sharon's care for the early years of her life. Thus, Sharon had initially been cared for primarily by her grandmother while her mother finished school and worked. Although she had lived with her mother for most of her grammar school and adolescent years, Sharon had frequently retreated to her grandmother's home in times of family conflict.

Treatment during Pregnancy

The first home-based session included two therapists, Sharon, Mrs. Smith, and a cousin who was emotionally supportive to Sharon. Sharon was often intimidated by her grandmother, an extremely talkative and forceful individual. In this first session, Sharon and her grandmother agreed that there were many conflicts in the family, and that it would be helpful to meet with the therapists once each week to discuss family problems and to prepare for the infant's arrival. Sharon was very nervous about this pregnancy and afraid that she would lose another baby. The grandmother was able to share that she had had several miscarriages herself and understood Sharon's concern. Thus, from the first session, the therapists facilitated more open and affect-laden communication between Sharon and her grandmother.

Sharon agreed to allow the therapists to refer her to a high-risk prenatal program and to assist her in keeping her appointments there. For the next few months, the treatment had two functions. The first was to help Sharon and her family understand and resolve some of their recurring conflicts, so that a more stable and supportive environment could be established for Sharon and her baby. The second function was to ensure that Sharon received the specialized prenatal care that she needed. The focus of the present discussion is on the family therapy, which addressed the first function of treatment. However, it should be understood that the efforts made by the therapists to support Sharon's medical care were viewed so positively by both Sharon and her family that these efforts were critical in attaining the trust needed to do the family work.

In the first weeks of treatment, which primarily involved Sharon and Mrs. Smith, some of the patterns and difficulties in this family became apparent. First of all, Sharon's mother, though invited, failed to come to the sessions, already demonstrating her reluctance to meet with both her mother and her daughter. Mrs. Smith dominated the sessions in spite of her granddaughter's attempts to talk. Mrs. Smith was accustomed to telling her family what to do and how to behave. She did not know how to listen. Also, one of the main foci of Mrs. Smith's discourse was extensive criticism of Sharon's boyfriend, Chris, the father of her unborn child. Mrs. Smith had "no use" for Chris; she accused him of not being able or willing to support Sharon. She talked of how the situation reminded her of Susan's pregnancy with Sharon. This alerted the therapists to an intergenerational or multigenerational transmission process: Mrs. Smith had had "no use" for Sharon's father, either. Sharon acknowledged never knowing her father and having no idea where he was now. With feeling, she said that she wanted her child to have a father, and so she wanted to keep Chris in her life.

In the second month of treatment, Sharon and her grandmother were already acknowledging somewhat improved communication. Mrs. Smith was beginning to listen to Sharon, although she still insisted that Sharon did not listen to her—which really meant that Sharon did not always do what she wanted. For a few sessions, one therapist talked with Mrs. Smith while the other talked alone with Sharon. This gave each an opportunity to tell her own story fully. This strategy was particularly helpful for Sharon, who began to talk more about her mother. It was clear by now that it was difficult for Sharon to say positive things about her mother in front of her grandmother, because these two women sometimes competed for the role of chief parent.

Over the next few sessions, Sharon continued to share that she had recently had some positive contact with her mother and wished to repair that relationship. Although Susan still did not attend therapy sessions, she and Sharon were seeing each other more often and with less accompanying conflict. However, Sharon told of being uncomfortable with her mother's present boyfriend, who was in his early 20s. The issue of her mother's relationships with men still troubled Sharon greatly.

By the end of the third month of treatment, Sharon was ready to deliver her baby and was planning to move back in with her mother after the birth. Although she and her grandmother were much more able to talk and listen to each other, there was some continuing conflict, especially over Chris. Sharon's mother had managed to avoid joining the treatment except in regard to very practical issues, such as planning medical appointments. Finally, in early January, Sharon delivered a healthy full-term baby girl, Christine, and returned home to her mother's apartment.

Sharon Becomes a Mother

Living with Susan, Sharon, and Christine were Sharon's 12-year-old half-sister, Dawn, and Susan's young boyfriend, Ray. Although sessions continued at Susan's apartment, Susan herself was seldom there. Efforts were made to accommodate her work schedule, but Susan continued to show some reluctance to join the treatment.

Conflict soon erupted in this situation, and Sharon again returned to her grandmother's. For the next few months of treatment, Sharon alternated between these two residences, with her mother caring for the baby when Sharon needed a break. Sharon, who was now close to 19 years of age, began to consider looking for her own place to live. Both her mother and her grandmother still objected to Chris, and Sharon felt that with these two strong women so firmly present in her life, she was losing control of her own baby. She wanted to be her child's primary caretaker and did not want to relinquish the care of Christine to either her mother or her grandmother. Finding a balance between taking advantage of the support these two offered in regard to the baby's care and maintaining her own role as mother became a focus of treatment.

Although much of the therapy during this interim period was carried out with Sharon alone, the focus of the work was on intergenerational family patterns. These patterns included women relinquishing their roles as mothers to their own mothers and women totally expelling male figures from relationships with their young children. Sharon began to acknowledge that there were some problems with Chris. She wanted him to get a job, and she felt he was not as strongly motivated as she to finish an education. But he did not abuse her, and he did try to maintain a relationship with her and their child. She wanted to continue to give him a chance and to encourage him to get on with education and job training. Sharon and Chris began to look actively for an independent living arrangement. During this whole period, Sharon remained in the alternative educational program and was working on her GED.

A Crisis

A period of crisis finally brought all the family issues into clearer focus for everyone. Mrs. Smith called one day to report great conflict in her home over Sharon and Chris. In an emergency session, Mrs. Smith shared that she felt she was reliving the earlier situation with her daughter Susan. She said that Sharon's father and Chris were both "dogs," and that she, Mrs. Smith, was reliving the anger and hurt she had experienced when her daughter would not "listen" to her. This was pointed out to Mrs. Smith as an example of the intergenerational projection process regarding men.

As Sharon's mother, Susan, began to feel more of the stress of caring for her daughter and her granddaughter, she also agreed to join family sessions. A few sessions included Mrs. Smith but most involved Susan alone with her two daughters, Sharon and Dawn. During these sessions, Susan revealed a family secret: She said that she was the only child in her family who had not been fathered by the "grandfather," Mr. Robert Smith. Susan did not learn this until she was an adult, although she had always felt that her parents favored her siblings. When she was little, she had been brought to visit a man who was never identified to her. She believed now that he was her father, although she and her mother had never discussed it. So Susan and Sharon actually shared the experience of not knowing their fathers and of feeling left out in their families. Acknowledging this history helped Susan accept Sharon's wish to keep Chris involved in her baby's life.

Another critical issue with which this family began to deal was Susan's lifestyle and its impact on her daughters. The two daughters, Sharon and Dawn, were both very critical of their mother's new young boyfriend and felt she was trying to be an adolescent like them. As Susan began to mourn her own lost adolescence, she recognized the effect her behavior had on her daughters. This also led her to become more responsive to Dawn's emerging adolescent needs. These two began to communicate much more openly and effectively, as Susan asserted her wish to care for Dawn in such a way as to prevent another intergenerational repetition of an adolescent pregnancy in this family.

Mother and Grandmother

Another important issue on which Susan and Sharon worked was the role of mother. Susan often wanted to take over the care of Christine, although she also resented that responsibility. Susan wanted the experience of finally being a successful parent, but at the same time she wanted to get on with her own life. Ways in which she could support and assist Sharon without taking over were explored. As Susan supported Sharon, she became proud that her daughter could really be a good mother. As she was able to let Sharon separate and be a mother, Susan began to enjoy her role as supportive grandmother. Susan also came to understand that if she took over the care of Christine, the family cycle would repeat itself, leading to parenting problems in future generations.

At the conclusion of treatment, many of these intergenerational issues had been resolved. Role conflicts and communication issues had been addressed. Chris had frequent contact with Christine, who was attached to both her parents and was developing well. Sharon was living on her own and attending school, with her family's encouragement and support. Susan, Sharon, and Dawn were communicating openly, and both girls were doing well in school and with their peers.

Discussion

The Smith family illustrates many of the intergenerational themes presented by families with teenage parents. The home-based family therapy approach used in this treatment involved many of the key family and extended family members, and allowed the multigenerational themes to be addressed directly. Many of the family therapy sessions focused on the relationships among the grandmother, the mother, and both daughters. It was clear that Sharon's pregnancy had evoked memories of prior adolescent pregnancies in the two previous generations of this family. As these issues were discussed openly in the family, communication between the generations was enhanced; role conflicts regarding the parenting and care of the baby were discussed; and the guilt and angry feelings of the past were separated from present events. The multiple generations of women in the family were helped to see that they were projecting their anger toward men in their past onto the baby's teenage father. The multigenerational family cycle of the exclusion of fathers was broken, as the teenage father was encouraged to maintain an active role in his child's life. Through this family therapy intervention, the teenage mother was supported by her family in becoming a competent parent, living on her own, and completing her education.

Summary

The Smith family can be seen as a prototype of many families with a history of intergenerational adolescent pregnancy. Their case illustrates the power of the home-based family therapy approach to build trust with families; to address multigenerational issues directly; and to produce positive change for teenage parents and their children.

CHILD SEXUAL ABUSE

Clinicians may discover a multigenerational pattern in families of children who have been referred for sexual abuse. According to Kagan and Schlossberg (1989), "Crisis oriented families typically act out themes which have never been resolved, e.g., the mother who was brutally raped at 13 finds her own daughters sexually abused at around the same age in a seemingly unstoppable cycle of multigenerational trauma" (p. 3). Clinicians should not automatically assume, however, that all cases of child sexual abuse are multigenerational in nature (Alexander, 1990; MacFarlane et al., 1986; Trepper & Barrett, 1986).

In recent years, as the denial about sexual abuse has begun to change to knowledge, incidence studies have begun to document the extent of the problem. Many experts in this area believe that the actual incidence of abuse greatly exceeds the reported statistics (Finkelhor, 1995; Finkelhor & Dziuba-Leatherman, 1994; Gil, 1995, 1996). For further discussions of clinical interventions in sexual abuse cases, therapists are referred to Gil (1995, 1996), MacFarlane et al. (1986), and Trepper and Barrett (1986).

The following case example illustrates some of the issues involved in multigenerational child sexual abuse, including the need for both individual and family work.

Case Example

Mary was the 7-year-old only child of Alice Duffy, a 35-year-old single parent from an Irish American family. Because Mary had become increasingly depressed and withdrawn, Mary's teacher became concerned and referred her to the school guidance counselor. In one of the early sessions with the counselor, Mary revealed to the counselor that she was afraid of her mother's boyfriend, Paul Graham (age 36). Mary became so frightened that she refused to say anything more about it for the remainder of the session. In Mary's next session, the guidance counselor told her that many children had told her that they were afraid of someone, and that often it was because they had hurt them in some way and warned them not to tell anyone about it. Mary then told the counselor that Paul had hurt her "tee-tee." When this was explored, it became clear that some form of sexual molestation had occurred. The counselor was bound by law to report this to child protective services.

Mary's mother, Alice, was called and asked to come to school. Although Mary had tried to tell her mother of the abuse, Alice had initially ignored her daughter's concerns. To Alice's credit, after the counselor met with her, she then supported her daughter and asked her boyfriend to leave her home. By the time Mary and her mother were referred to the sexual abuse treatment unit, Mary had already received a medical exam; child protective services had removed her from the home and placed her in a foster home while they conducted their investigation; and the boyfriend was facing criminal charges as a result of the sexual abuse.

The therapist's first meeting was with the mother alone in her home while Mary was still in foster care. Alice reported that she had asked child protective services to return Mary to her home, as she had "thrown Paul out" and he had been arrested and was under the jurisdiction of the courts for his sexual abuse of Mary. She also tearfully reported that she was feeling very guilty for not having protected and believed her daughter from the start. The therapist obtained written permission from Alice to contact all of the agencies involved: Mary's school, child protective services, the foster family, the police, and the prosecutor's office. She sent a letter to each agency requesting information, and then followed up with phone calls.

The therapist next met alone with Mary, who was brought to her office by the child protective service worker. (This session was held in the therapist's office in order to protect Mary's privacy.) The therapist used this session to join with Mary and to begin to explore the sexual abuse. Anatomically correct dolls and drawings were available. Mary reported that while her mother was out shopping, Paul came into Mary's room as she was napping and began touching her "tee-tee." When asked to point to this on an anatomically correct drawing, she pointed to the vaginal area. She reported that he first touched her with his finger and then with his "pee-pee." When asked to point this out on the drawing, she pointed to his penis. She stated that he pushed his "pee-pee" in and it hurt. (This was consistent with the medical report the therapist had obtained.) When asked what happened next, Mary said she ran to the bathroom, locked the door, and stayed there until she heard her mother's voice. The therapist praised her for thinking to do this. Mary then told her mother that Paul had touched her "tee-tee." Her mother then went into the bedroom with Paul. They had a loud argument, but this was never mentioned again.

The therapist continued home sessions with the mother, while conducting office sessions with Mary to give her the privacy unavailable in her foster home. In one home visit with the mother, Alice told the therapist that the experience Mary had been through had stirred up a great deal for her. As a young girl of 10, Alice had been sexually abused by her father. She had told her mother, who did not believe her. Alice cried as she told this story, and asked over and over, "How could I not believe my own daughter?" and "How could I let this happen?" When the therapist asked Alice how she might answer those questions, she cried and said she "did not want to lose Paul." Mary's father had abandoned her when she became pregnant; both of her parents had died; and she was afraid of being alone. She also missed Paul's financial contributions to the household. The therapist told Alice that she understood her feelings, and encouraged her to use some of their sessions to explore these issues further. The therapist also reinforced her decision to remove Paul from her home and to support her daughter now.

Approximately 1 week after this session, Mary was returned to her mother's home. When Alice brought Mary to her next session, the therapist first met with them together and then divided the rest of the session to give Mary and Alice each some individual time. In the portion of the session in which both were in the room, Mary seemed timid and withdrawn with her mother. The therapist sensed that they were holding back from each other.

Mary was seen alone first, and the therapist asked her how she felt being with her mother. She replied, "Scared," and began to cry. When the therapist inquired about why she felt scared, she said that she thought her mother was "mad" at her because she had "told on Paul." When the therapist explored further why she felt this, she said, "My mom did not believe me at first." The therapist asked what Mary hoped would happen now between her and her mother; she tearfully stated, "She'll love me again." The therapist told Mary that she sensed that Mary very much wanted her mother's love. Mary nodded. The therapist asked whether Mary would accept some help from her in talking to her mother about this. Mary eagerly agreed. The therapist asked her permission to share some of Mary's concerns with her mother. Mary hesitated at first but then agreed.

While the therapist spoke with Alice alone, Mary played in the waiting room. The therapist first asked Alice what she felt during the session together. Alice reported, "It felt strange. We seem so far apart." She later explained that this was not a new feeling for her, as there had often been distance between them in the past. The therapist then told Alice that Mary had felt that distance also, and that she had Mary's permission to share her concerns. She explained to the mother that Mary was afraid that her mother would be mad at her for making Paul go away. Alice cried and said that she had been at first, but she was not angry with her now and only wanted to help her daughter. The therapist asked whether Alice would be willing to talk with Mary about this. She agreed.

Mary was brought back into the session, and she took a chair closer to her mother. The therapist moved her chair close to both of them and told Mary that she had shared her concerns with her mother. The therapist next asked Alice to talk to her daughter about this. Alice blurted out, "I'm not mad at you, Mary." She then started crying. Mary began crying too. The therapist moved their chairs closer together and encouraged them to hold each other. Mary moved from her chair and eagerly went into her mother's arms. The therapist quietly encouraged Alice to tell Mary of her love for her. She did so; Mary then said, "I thought you would be mad at me." Alice replied hesitantly, "I was at first, but I'm not now." She added, "I just wish that I had believed you before." The therapist asked the mother whether she believed Mary now. The mother replied, "Absolutely." The therapist asked her to explain to Mary that she believed her and to ask her forgiveness for not believing her earlier.

The therapist asked that they continue to meet in her office, and said that in the next session she would give them each some time alone and then meet with them together. In the next few sessions, Mary played out her anger at Paul, but was not yet ready to address her anger at her mother for not believing her. She used the family doll figures to beat up on the male doll and throw him angrily in the toy box. This continued for a number of sessions.

In her individual sessions, Alice talked more about her own sexual abuse experience and about her anger at both her mother and her father. These feelings were explored over a number of sessions. The "together time" was used during this period to find bonding activities that Mary and her mother could pursue together. Alice was encouraged to read to her daughter during this part of each session. Initially, they both sat rigidly in their chairs. The therapist encouraged them to try the "homework task" of reading together at bedtime. Gradually, they seemed closer in the "together" part of the session.

Finally, after 2 months, Alice stated that she was ready to tell Mary what had happened to her as a child and to let her know how bad she felt that "history was repeating itself." Mary listened avidly as her mother described her experiences.

In the next session together, Alice went on to share with her daughter how angry she had been at her own father for abusing her. The therapist helped Alice to ask whether Mary had been angry at Paul. Mary nodded timidly, and then moved to the toy area and began shoving the male doll angrily in the toy box. The therapist encouraged Alice to join Mary on the floor in the play area. Both of them happily played out their anger at the male doll. They both left the session more animated than the therapist had ever seen them.

It took much longer (3 months) for Mary to begin to address her anger at her mother. During this time, the therapist began to alternate weekly sessions between the office, which continued to follow the individual and "together time" format, and with home-based sessions where they worked on the bonding between Mary and her mother. In the home-based sessions, the therapist helped them to establish a special "cuddle time" just before bedtime, in which they would cuddle together and Alice would read to Mary. Initially, they were awkward as this was role-played on the couch in the living room, but gradually they seemed more at ease.

In the individual sessions in the office, Mary continued to play out the abuse and began to draw pictures. At first the little girl was very small in the bottom quarter of the page. Mary was encouraged to tell stories about her drawings. She told how the little girl was a "bad girl" because she let the "bad man" touch her. (This feeling that she was responsible for Paul's actions is a very common reaction among child victims of sexual abuse.) The therapist asked Mary what she thought she did. Mary cried and said, "I smiled at him." The therapist told Mary that she had a beautiful smile and that her smile did not cause this to happen to her. The therapist explained that it was Paul's fault, not hers, and that any time an adult abuses a little girl it is never the child's fault. In later sessions, Mary began to describe the ways in which Paul had threatened to hurt her if she ever talked to her mother about the incident again. (This intimidation is also quite common among perpetrators of child sexual abuse.) The therapist helped Mary to see that she was just a scared little girl who had done the best she could do at the time. Over the months, Mary's mood and affect began to change.

Eventually, in her individual sessions, Alice began addressing her own anger at her mother for not believing and protecting her. After a number of these sessions, Alice asked, "I wonder if Mary feels the same way toward me." In their next "together time," Alice asked Mary whether she remembered the time when they discussed how her mother had also been sexually abused by her father. Mary nodded. Alice asked whether she remembered their talk about how angry she was at her father. Again Mary nodded. Alice then told her that she had also been very angry at her mother, who also did not believe her or protect her. With the therapist's help, Alice said to Mary, "I am sure that you had some angry feelings toward me." Mary was silent and looked fearfully at the therapist. With the therapist's prompting, Alice explained to Mary that if she did have those angry feelings, she (Alice) would not be mad at her (Mary). Mary nodded and cried. The mother spontaneously put her arms around Mary and told her that she understood her anger and wanted her to know that she loved her. Mary did not speak much in this session, but continued to hold her mother.

This session was a turning point for Mary and Alice. Mary spontaneously invited her mother during the next home-based session to play "doll babies" with her. They spent an enjoyable time "feeding" and "cuddling" the "baby." Their relationship continued to improve, and treatment was terminated 2 months later.

Discussion

This case illustrates many lessons for family therapists and workers. This family's crisis clearly demonstrates how several outside agencies (including child protective services, the school, medical authorities, the police, etc.) quickly became involved in the crisis (Alexander, 1990; MacFarlane et al., 1986; Trepper & Barrett, 1986).

The therapist flexibly utilized the multisystems model in her combination of treatment modalities. In this case, because of the mother's own sexual abuse history, individual work with her was necessary. In order to allow both Mary and Alice the privacy to explore their issues individually, many sessions were conducted in the therapist's office rather than in the home. This is very important in cases such as these, where a child's natural sense of trust has been destroyed and needs to be rebuilt.

The therapist began building the bond between parent and child gradually through sessions together in her office. Only after preliminary work in this area had been done and more trust had been established were home-based sessions resumed. These were carefully alternated with office-based sessions so that the individual work could be done with some degree of privacy.

JUVENILE DELINQUENCY

As discussed throughout this chapter, a crisis involving an adolescent may be a repetition of a trauma suffered by a parent that has never been openly discussed. The following case illustrates the ways in which themes of secrets about father absence and delinquency or criminal behavior can be repeated through many crises in the family. It is also an excellent example of the ways in which prior losses or traumas can become "toxic secrets" (Boyd-Franklin, 1989, 1993; Imber-Black, 1993; Kagan & Schlossberg, 1989) that are never discussed.

Case Example

Aisha Simmons, a 30-year-old African American single mother, was referred for family treatment by the police following her 14-year-old son Malik's second arrest for juvenile delinquent activity. His first arrest had been for defacing subway cars with graffiti. He had been referred for family therapy as a result of the first arrest; his mother had brought him to the first session, but he refused to return. Malik's second arrest, approximately 1 month prior to the current referral, was for "joyriding" with two boys who had stolen a car. This pattern was becoming a repetitive one for him: Each crisis was triggered by Malik's following other adolescents into committing acts of serious delinquent behavior.

In the first session of mandated therapy following the second arrest, Aisha was extremely angry and critical of Malik. She described him repeatedly as "bad," and reported that he had hurt her so much that she was giving up on him and had therefore "shut him out." She stated that she was very "disappointed in him." The therapist initially felt overwhelmed by Aisha, for a number of reasons. She was very argumentative, often contradicting statements made by the therapist. Her tone of voice and body language in the session often appeared angry or hostile; she would roll her eyes, suck her teeth, and shake her head as the therapist spoke. Aisha also talked incessantly, and it was very difficult for the therapist to intervene. In addition, the therapist was troubled by the fact that each time he asked the mother about the family history or attempted to construct a family tree or genogram (Boyd-Franklin, 1989; McGoldrick & Gerson, 1985), she either changed the topic or said, "That's the past; I leave it in the past." In short, the therapist felt dismissed by the mother and felt that she scapegoated her son constantly. After the first session, the therapist attended supervision and was helped to process some of his own feelings of anger at the mother.

With the supervisor's help, the therapist joined with Aisha. Information emerged slowly during the first months of treatment, as Aisha very gradually began to share some of her own history. Her mother had died when she was 3 years old, and she had been sent to live with her maternal grandmother and aunt. Her father had remarried and had four sons, whom she did not know well. She felt abandoned by her father. Moreover, the therapist began to understand Aisha's intense fears for and anger at Malik as he learned that Aisha also felt abandoned by Malik's father, who had been incarcerated since Malik was 1 year old. (This had been kept secret from Malik, who had been told that his father was dead.) It now became clear that the repeated crises with Malik and the police reflected a pattern in the family, and that Aisha was terrified that he would "follow in his father's footsteps."

The therapist could now empathize with Aisha's response to Malik. Behind the facade of anger lay her intense fears for him, including that he would be the third "man" in her life to abandon her if he were sent to prison like his father. As these themes emerged, the therapist began to talk to Aisha about sharing these secrets with Malik. She resisted. In addition to meeting with Aisha and Malik, the therapist also joined them for a number of sessions at the school and with Malik's probation officer, and accompanied the family to court.

Finally, Malik created another crisis: He was again caught joyriding in a stolen car. His mother was furious. During the session, she conveyed a great deal of anger at Malik, as well as at the therapist for not "fixing" him. Eventually, however, the therapist helped Aisha to see the importance of discussing with Malik her fears for him and his father's history.

In the first of a very emotional series of sessions, Aisha told Malik about his father's incarceration. Malik, angry at first, began to ask questions about his father. Aisha adamantly opposed Malik's request to contact his father. After many sessions, she relented as far as allowing Malik to write his father a letter.

In a later session, Aisha, with the therapist's help, shared her genogram with Malik. He seemed fascinated by her father's large family, of whom Malik had had very little knowledge. Because of her feelings of abandonment and fears that the members of this family would judge her parenting of Malik, Aisha was reluctant to let Malik contact them.

As sessions continued, Aisha's earlier statement that when Malik began to get in trouble she had "shut him out" began to make sense. She had learned through many painful experiences with men that "when they hurt, disappoint, or abandon you, you shut them out." Finally, she was able to listen to Malik's feelings of being shut out by her. His crises had served the function of pulling her back into his life.

Aisha was able to make a firm contract with Malik about continued attendance at family sessions, school performance, and adhering to the terms of his probation. She learned new communication and problem-solving skills, and she began to praise him more for small changes. For the first time, she worked on consistent disciplinary measures. She enforced his curfew and established clear consequences for his behavior. As a result, Malik's behavior began to improve. The crises decreased and finally stopped. He passed the school year and was promoted to the next grade. Family sessions ended after he successfully completed his probation. The therapist conducted brief monthly "booster sessions" (Bry & Krinsley, 1992) by phone with Aisha and Malik for 3 months to make sure that the positive behavior continued.

DRUG OR ALCOHOL ABUSE

Adolescent drug or alcohol abuse is a particularly disturbing presenting problem because it places teens at risk for many dangerous consequences, including overdoses, HIV/AIDS through needle sharing, crime, and violence. Moreover, adolescents often pay for their drug habits by shoplifting, prostitution, and dealing drugs to others, which put the adolescents even more at risk. As is the case with gang activity, adolescents are often introduced to alcohol and drug use by "hanging around with the wrong crowd."

Adolescents with family histories involving parental alcohol or drug abuse are often more vulnerable to addiction themselves and are frequently raised by grandparents. These grandparents may be struggling with their own guilt about their substance abuse histories, their feelings that they failed as parents because of their adult children's addiction, and their strong desire to "save the grandchildren" from a similar pattern.

Many grandparents have been given custody of their grandchildren when child protective services interceded with the courts to mandate removal of the children from the homes of their biological parents. Despite such formal custody arrangements, the biological parents may still be in and out of the grandparents' homes, which can prove very disruptive. Sometimes the adolescents' behavior is modeled after that of their parents, and the older family members have difficulty setting limits on their adult children's behavior. The following case illustrates these dynamics.

Case Example

Ramon, a 16-year-old Puerto Rican adolescent, was referred for family treatment by the court after his arrest for possession of marijuana in school. The Ramos family consisted of Ms. Melinda Ramos (age 65), his paternal grandmother; his younger sister, Maria (age 12); his father, Arturo (age 40), who was in and out of the family and had a long history of drug abuse; and his young uncle, Pablo (age 25), who worked in a nearby car wash. Ramon's mother had died in a car crash when he was 3.

The court mandated that the family receive home-based treatment. Ms. Ramos and Ramon were present for the first session, and Maria wandered in and out. Ms. Ramos had been unaware of Ramon's drug involvement and asked him many questions about his activities. At first he was very surly and refused to talk about these issues. The session took place in the kitchen (where all major family activities seemed to occur). Ms. Ramos chopped onions and garlic at the table during the session, and stirred pots on the stove throughout.

This first session focused on the immediate issues for Ramon, including his suspension from school and his pending court hearing. With the therapist's encouragement, Ms. Ramos, who was obviously the family spokesperson and the "switchboard" through which all communication occurred in the family, approached the school and helped to arrange for his return to an alternative school, where he would have more individualized attention.

During a later home-based session, Ramon's young uncle, Pablo, returned early from work and came into the house. The therapist invited him to sit at the table. Ms. Ramos offered him something to eat and drink. As the session progressed, it was clear that Ramon really looked up to Pablo. The therapist asked Pablo to ask Ramon about how he had first gotten involved in drug use. Ramon explained that he had been recruited by drug dealers at age 11 to act as a "runner," selling "nickel bags" (small $5 packets) of marijuana and, later, cocaine to his friends at school. He did not use drugs himself at first, but as he got more involved in dealing, he began to smoke marijuana and later to snort cocaine. Once he developed a drug habit, his dealing accelerated to support his addiction. With his grandmother's encouragement, Pablo talked with Ramon about how he had been on a path similar to Ramon's, but how he had gotten help and "pulled himself back." He spoke to a very resistant Ramon about getting drug treatment. Pablo also revealed Ramon's father's drug history for the first time to the therapist. Ms. Ramos, who was very troubled by her oldest son's drug addiction, refused to talk about it initially.

In the meantime, Ramon presented another crisis: A house where he was hanging out was raided by the police, and everyone inside was arrested for drug possession. Ms. Ramos called the therapist in a panic. When the therapist made a home visit, he discovered Ramon's father, Arturo, in the living room. He had returned from drug treatment and was staying in the family home. The therapist spent a few minutes getting to know Arturo and asked whether he was aware of what was happening with Ramon. Arturo replied that he knew only that Ramon had been arrested. The therapist asked Ms. Ramos to share the details with Arturo. The therapist then told Arturo that he was one of the most important people in Ramon's life, and asked for his support in helping his son. Arturo looked skeptical but agreed to participate in sessions.

In the next session, Arturo and Pablo supported Ms. Ramos's attempts to set limits for Ramon. They all agreed to a curfew and to clear consequences if it was violated. The next week, in a very moving session, Arturo was able to share with Ramon his own history of drug addiction and dealing. He told Ramon that he did not want him to turn out "like me." He also told Ramon about his drug treatment program, and Ramon listened intently but refused to go.

Finally, a week later, Ramon created still another crisis: He was arrested again, and this time he was placed in a juvenile detention center. The therapist first met with Ramon at the center, and then went to the home for a family session with Ms. Ramos, Arturo, and Pablo. She discussed with them the need for "tough love," in which they would request that the court mandate drug treatment in a locked facility for Ramon. Ms. Ramos was appalled at first. She repeated, "*No, el es mi bambino*" ("No, he is my baby"). She wanted to ask the judge to release Ramon to her custody. The therapist asked Arturo and Pablo to discuss this with Ms. Ramos. Arturo reminded her that she had bailed him out as an adolescent and repeatedly since. Ms. Ramos became a bit defensive and replied, *"Pero el es mi familia"* ("But he is my family"). This was true to her Latino culture; love of family was all-important to her. The therapist then asked the "miracle" question (Berg, 1994). That is, she asked what she would want to see happen for Ramon if a miracle occurred during the night. Ms. Ramos replied that she would like to see him "turn his life around." The therapist asked her what she meant by that. She described wanting him to "finish school, get a job, lead a good life." The therapist asked whether Ms. Ramos knew someone who had "turned his life around." She thought for a long time and then turned to Pablo and said, "You did." He seemed surprised.

The therapist asked Pablo what he thought about what his mother had said. He said he had never thought of his life in that way. The therapist asked his mother to describe what she meant by "turned his life around." Ms. Ramos described a time when Pablo was about 16 and was in and out of trouble with the law and drugs. He was arrested, and a judge ordered him to a drug detox program and a treatment facility. Pablo reported that he worked with a counselor there and had been involved in a Twelve-Step program (Narcotics Anonymous) since. The therapist commended him for turning his life around, and then asked him how Ms. Ramos and the family had supported him in this process. Pablo said, "She never gave up on me." Ms. Ramos was in tears.

The therapist faced two difficult decisions. She wanted to validate Ms. Ramos's love and caring, but to address her enabling and co-dependency. At the same time, she did not want to leave Arturo out by artificially setting Pablo up as the "good son." The therapist therefore turned to Ms. Ramos and said, "So you went along with the judge and still continued to support your son. What stopped you from trying to get the judge to let him out?" She replied, "It was helping him."

The therapist then included Arturo and asked what he was thinking about what had been said. He hesitated and then turned to his mother and said, "I wish you had done that for me." He explained that his mother had always talked the judges, police, and school authorities out of punishing him. The therapist tried to reframe this by saying, "So you knew your mother loved you, but you wished she could have used more 'tough love.'" Arturo said, "Yes." The therapist asked Arturo what he wanted for his son. He said, "For him to be clean of drugs." The therapist asked him to talk to his mother about this. In a very passionate discussion, both Arturo and Pablo emphasized that Ms. Ramos was a loving mother and grandmother, and that they all needed to have "tough love" now in order to get Ramon the help he needed. Ms. Ramos tearfully agreed.

In the next session, the therapist discussed with Ms. Ramos, Arturo, and Pablo the possibility of doing an "intervention" (Treadway, 1989) with Ramon at the juvenile detention facility. She rehearsed with them the process of having a session with Ramon in which they would all tell him of their love and each express their fears for him if he continued on his present path. In order to empower Arturo, the therapist asked him to call the counselor at the juvenile detention center and his probation officer and ask for a meeting.

A family session was held at the juvenile detention center that included Ramon, Pablo, Arturo, Ms. Ramos, the therapist, the juvenile detention counselor, and the probation officer. All of the family members told Ramon of their love and stressed that he must get help. In a very large step, Ms. Ramos told him that with his father and uncle's support, she was going to ask the judge to mandate drug treatment for him. Ramon initially was angry and resistant, but also seemed quite surprised by this turn of events. Finally, the probation officer reported that Ramon's choices were few. If he did not decide to report for drug treatment, the judge might decide, because of his age, to treat him as an adult and send him to the main adult prison. Ramon looked frightened by this and asked what was involved in drug treatment. The therapist asked his father to discuss this with Ramon, who agreed by the end of the session to enter drug treatment.

About 3 days later, on the court date, the entire family appeared to support the "tough love" position of mandated drug treatment.

DISCUSSION

As can be seen in these case examples, even families facing seemingly intractable multigenerational problems can be aided by trained family workers to recognize the causes of their pain and to begin, with help, not to let their past dictate their future. The pitfall for family workers is to ignore patterns of repetitive crises and attempt to "fix" each problem as it arises. This may, in fact, exacerbate a family's situation as the members unconsciously increase their acting-out behaviors.

CHAPTER 5

Working with Children and Their Families

This chapter provides an overview of the benefits of home-based therapy for families with young children. We begin by highlighting the importance of identifying family resources; this can be particularly useful for parents of young children. The chapter then provides techniques for working with parents, showing how home-based sessions can be used to support and enhance skills needed in daily life. The chapter concludes with three sections describing and illustrating home-based work with families of infants, preschool children, and school-age children.

Many of the techniques described here have been used in home-based programs (Henggeler et al., 1998; Tatum et al., 1995) that have been shown in several studies to be effective means of intervention with at-risk families (see Chapter 10).

IDENTIFYING FAMILY RESOURCES

Knowledge of the resources in a particular neighborhood or community can help a clinician empower a family to obtain good child care. Such resources may include after-school monitoring for the child of a working parent, a church with a mentoring and tutoring program, concerned friends and neighbors, or various community programs and agencies. Assessing and utilizing these multisystemic strengths can have a profound impact on a child and family and can result in the provision of needed support (Henggeler et al., 1998).

Children who are most at risk include those living in families where there is a history of proven or alleged abuse or neglect, and those living in very isolated family units with few supports. With at-risk infants and young children, their safety, well-being, and protection are primary. Clinicians should not assume that biological parents are primarily responsible for raising their children, especially when these parents are very young. In many cultural groups, family or extended family members may have decisive roles in child rearing. It is therefore important to consider the possibility of multiple parental figures or surrogate parents. This can become particularly important when a child's biological parents are unable to care for him or her.

Case Example: A Home for Honey

Honey was a 2-month-old African American baby girl. She had been hospitalized since her premature birth, and her mother, a 20-year-old cocaine addict, had abandoned her after checking out of the hospital. Because of Honey's initial medical condition, including fetal drug addiction and congenital heart problems, she had remained in the hospital for longer than usual. She was absolutely adorable and became a favorite of the nurses and doctors, receiving a great deal of attention from them.

Violet Parker, an African American caseworker with child protective services who had been assigned to Honey shortly after her birth, was also very taken with this lovely, responsive baby and determined to find a good foster home for her. Because of Honey's fragile medical condition, the worker sought a home able to provide specialized medical care to infants. Honey was released to such a home approximately 2 months after her birth. The foster parents were an older couple who, despite "falling in love" with Honey, were unable to adopt her.

Child protective services were required by state law either to return Honey to her biological family through a reunification process or to find an adoptive family for her. The child protective services worker located the biological mother's family through her contacts in the community, but Honey's mother was unwilling to seek drug treatment and work toward reunification. Honey's biological grandmother would have adopted Honey, were it not for her own serious medical condition. The grandmother assisted the worker in locating other family members who might be able to care for Honey.

The grandmother helped the worker construct a genogram of extended family members and close family friends. This process resulted in the discovery of a family member—the grandmother's niece, Marilyn—who desperately wanted a child. Marilyn (age 35), and her husband, John, had been discussing the possibility of adoption, as they could not have children of their own. With Honey's grandmother's help, Marilyn and John were contacted. A meeting was arranged in which the couple spent the day visiting with Honey at the grandmother's house. The worker, who transported Honey to this meeting and participated in this process, was delighted to see the immediate positive response of Honey to Marilyn and John, and vice versa. The couple decided to begin the process of petitioning to adopt Honey.

Discussion

This case had a very positive outcome because of the dedication and skills of the family worker. Her knowledge of the multisystems process and her awareness of the family's cultural strengths enabled her to reach out and locate extended family members who could intervene and adopt this child.

WORKING WITH PARENTS

Although a multisystemic perspective is essential, family therapists also need particular skills for working collaboratively with parents. This is especially important for parents of young children. Many mothers and fathers have never learned age-appropriate parenting skills. Problematic parenting may include inconsistent, permissive, authoritarian, neglectful, or abusive styles (Henggeler et al., 1998). These issues must be assessed early in the treatment process. As already discussed, the best strategy for observing these behaviors is visiting in the family's home. If this is not possible, the clinician can engage the family in role-playing or enacting (Minuchin, 1974) behaviors in an office-based session. There are many ways of working with parents. Here we address three: joining and therapeutic confrontation; behavioral parent training; and structural and systems interventions. The home-based practitioner may want to consider using a combination of all three of these methods, since each addresses a particular facet of the parent–child relationship.

As we have emphasized throughout this book, it is extremely important for the therapist to provide positive reinforcement by emphasizing the parents' strengths and the things that they are doing well. The therapist also becomes the "receptacle of hope" for the family. Often parents (and teachers) may have begun to despair. The therapist holds the belief in the possibility of change until the family can believe in it also. Henggeler et al. (1998) call this a "can-do attitude" (p. 30).

Joining and Therapeutic Confrontation

Many parents may be embarrassed by the behavior of their children and may have been judged by schools and other referral sources. Parents who feel judged will, in turn, be judgmental of their children. Earlier it was stated that clinicians may have difficulty joining with and maintaining an alliance with these parents, because they often speak angrily toward their children and scapegoat them in sessions (Haley, 1976; Minuchin, 1974). Parents may also, in their frustration, reject clinicians' help, particularly in the initial stages of treatment. It is important that clinicians avoid taking this response personally.

It is here that a therapist's "use of self" is so essential. A clinician should look for "something to like" in a parent and reframe the parent's behavior in a positive way. For example, extremely critical behavior can be reframed as "wanting the best for your son and pushing him to become the best he can be." Overprotective behavior can be reframed as "loving your daughter too much" (Aponte, 1995). It is essential that therapists emphasize positive parenting practices as much as possible (Henggeler et al., 1998). As clinicians and supervisors, we cannot overstate the importance of assessing a child's, a parent's, or a family's strengths. For example, a child who is not doing well in school may have a number of positive peers and excellent social skills. A parent may truly love his or her child, may be willing to "go the extra mile" to try to help this child, and be a good systems advocate on the child's behalf. A family may have lots of affection and a strong support network of extended family, friends, neighbors, "church family," etc.) (Henggeler et al., 1998).

There are times, however, when it is necessary to challenge parents—particularly when parental behavior may lead to abuse or neglect of a child. Challenging parents should not lead to unnecessary negative confrontations (Henggeler et al., 1998). It is never helpful, as indicated in Chapter 3, to get involved in an angry confrontation or screaming match. This can only destroy the therapeutic alliance and negate the opportunity for help. When therapeutic confrontations are necessary, the emphasis should be on the word "therapeutic." The following case example illustrates how a confrontation with a parent was framed into a caring intervention by the therapist.

Case Example

Ms. Charlotte Willis was an active drug addict, currently snorting heroin and abusing alcohol. She had gone through a brief period of recovery, during which the therapist had been able to address positive parenting practices with her and her three children—Gregory (age 11), Walter (age 9), and William (age 6). A failed love relationship led to a relapse. Once she began using drugs again, her oldest son, Gregory, was picked up by the police for shoplifting in a local store. Her youngest son, William, began acting out in school and was in danger of failing the year. When

William "talked back" to her, Ms. Willis hit him repeatedly in an angry outburst. A teacher noticed the bruises and reported Ms. Willis to child protective services. After an investigation, the children were removed and placed in foster care.

Ms. Willis was devastated and began using drugs more heavily. In a session with her family therapist, she expressed remorse, sorrow, and guilt for her abuse of her son. She asked the therapist's help in regaining custody of her children.

The therapist, in consultation with her supervisor, decided to engage in a therapeutic confrontation with her. Building on their relationship, she was careful first to acknowledge the love Ms. Willis had for her children and her attempts to be a good mother to them. The therapist praised her for the hard work on parenting strategies she had demonstrated in therapy. The therapist then confronted her directly with the reality of her drug use and the need for change. She said the following:

"Ms. Willis, you and I have worked together for a number of months, and I've seen how much you love your children and want them back. It's because I care about you and your children that I've got to be very 'real' and straight with you. I've seen you when you are not using drugs and alcohol and when you're high. To be honest, you are two different people. When you're sober, you are a loving mother; when you're high, the kids become an irritation, and you can hurt them very badly.

"I feel that I have to level with you. The only way that you will be able to get your children back is to voluntarily go into a drug detox and rehab program, and then seriously work a Twelve-Step and aftercare program to stay sober. You may not be ready to hear this yet. You may need to let your drug use leave you homeless or lose permanent custody of your kids before you get help. If you can convince me that you really want the help, then I'll 'go to the wall' with you and get you a program. If not, truly, you may not be able to get your kids back. When you're ready, you can get the help, but you have to take the first step."

Ms. Willis burst into tears and agreed to go to a detox and rehab program. The therapist acted immediately to facilitate that referral.

Discussion

Notice that this therapeutic confrontation was a gentle one, framed within the positive caring of a therapeutic relationship. The realities of Mrs. Willis's situation were made very clear to her, but this was done in a concerned and empathetic manner. Therapists are advised to seek supervision in such difficult cases, in order to avoid the very human response of becoming judgmental and punitive toward these parents.

Parent Training

There are many models of behavioral parent training (Dishion & Patterson, 1996; Eyberg, 1988; Forehand & McMahon, 1981; Sanders & Dadds, 1993; Webster-Stratton, 1993). Munger (1993) has, however, identified three general rules that clinicians can utilize in helping parents develop positive discipline and parenting practices:

1. First, the parent must learn to set clearly defined rules for the child's behavior.
2. Second, parents must develop sets of consequences that are inextricably linked to the rules. That is, when a child complies with the rule, positive reinforcement occurs; when a child does not comply, a negative consequence (i.e. punishment) occurs.
3. Third, parents must learn to effectively monitor a child's compliance or noncompliance with rules, even when the child is not in the parent's presence. (Munger, 1993, as quoted in Henggeler et al., 1998, p. 90)

Each of these strategies can be challenging for parents. When two parents are involved, both should agree on the rules and should enforce them consistently. It is also important to define the expected behavior clearly and specifically, so that anyone else (a babysitter, grandparent, older sibling, etc.) can tell whether the behavior has occurred. This will help to ensure that rules are enforced 100% of the time.

The rules should be explained clearly to a child, and ideally should be posted in a public place in the home (e.g., the refrigerator door). They should always be stated in terms of positive behaviors (e.g., "Jim will be inside the house at 6 P.M. on school nights," as opposed to "Jim will not be late"), and enforced in a clear, unemotional manner (Henggeler et al., 1998).

Munger (1993) and Henggeler et al. (1998) also stress the need for therapists to clarify for parents the strategies in designing rewards and punishments. Henggeler et al. (1998) state, "To be effective, the punishment must be experienced as aversive by the child and the reward must be highly desired" (p. 91). Many parents "give away" important rewards, such as snacks, desserts, TV time, video games, or special trips to McDonald's and Burger King, without realizing that these can be powerful positive reinforcers and rewards for their children.

Because the third guideline above applies to effectively monitoring school behavior as well as a child's after-school behavior without parental supervision, this is a particularly difficult aspect of parental work. There is a vast population of "latchkey children" who, from a very young age, are left without parental supervision from the time the children arrive home from school until 6:00, 7:00, or 8:00 P.M.. Parents with financial resources can pay for a babysitter, a tutor, or an after-school program. For many of the poor families who are referred for treatment, particularly in inner-city areas, such after-school supports are unobtainable.

In these circumstances, knowledge of the multisystemic options and resources—those available in the family, extended family, school, neighborhood, church, and community—is extremely important. Therapists should brainstorm with families about possible resources. There may be a grandmother, grandfather, or great-aunt who is retired and can provide help. If a mother is empowered to ask, churches often have many resources, including tutors, mentors, other volunteers, and after-school programs. A neighbor may be willing to check on the children, settle them into doing their homework, and provide a snack before a parent arrives home. With older children, parents often establish a phone check-in time, during which the children's plans for the afternoon are reviewed and discussed. Unfortunately, many overburdened parents neglect this monitoring function. Even when they are present in the home, they may be so overwhelmed that they retreat to their room and do not ask their children about homework and school assignments.

Once a clinician has inquired about a family's situation, including after-school arrangements and the flexibility (or lack thereof) of the parents' schedule after the school day, the clinician and family can develop more realistic plans in partnership. Within this partnership, the clinician can provide ideas for making, reinforcing, and monitoring rules, and can gradually empower the family to pursue them. (More information on behavioral strategies for parents is provided in Chapter 6.)

Structural and Systems Interventions

Minuchin (1974) has stressed the importance of helping parents to be "in charge" of their families and to assume an appropriate parental or executive role. If this does not occur, children become confused and begin to act out. Sometimes the problem is a disagreement between the parental figures on such issues as household rules or appropriate behavior for home and school. This can lead to inconsistent parenting practices. For example, a mother and father who are having difficulties in their own relationship may give conflicting messages to a child. A mother may be overinvolved with her son or daughter, while the father remains peripheral. In this case, it is important first to connect the peripheral parent to the child, and then to work on resolving the issues that have kept the parents from working together as a parental (executive) unit.

As illustrated earlier, sometimes the parental figures are members of the extended family. In some African American families, for example, a mother and a grandmother may share parenting responsibilities. Often in such a case, the mother first became a parent as a teenager. When a mother is 15 or 16, the grandmother of the baby may assume the parental role. In some families, the developmental transition of the mother's beginning to assume more appropriate parental responsibilities may not occur. More frequently, however, as the mother matures, she may begin to assume more parental responsibilities. In this process, conflicts can arise between "Grandma's rules" and "Mom's rules." Faced with this scenario, children begin to manipulate the adults and to act out. In this case, the therapist has the challenge of helping these family members to renegotiate their relationship so that they can work together more effectively as a parental or an executive unit and give clear, consistent messages to the children (Boyd-Franklin, 1989; Minuchin, 1974).

INFANTS

Reasons for Intervention

Babies and parents at risk are often targeted through their medical doctors. The reasons for intervention vary. Some programs focus on teenage parents; others target families in which there has been a history of abuse and/or neglect. Programs for at-risk babies may focus on infants with fetal drug or alcohol syndrome, failure-to-thrive infants, infants who initially test HIV-positive, or medically challenged babies and toddlers with congenital defects or developmental disabilities.

Although the infants are the initial presenting concern in these cases, the focus may quickly shift to concern about parents if there is evidence of serious problems, such as drug or alcohol addiction; HIV/AIDS, cancer, or another terminal illness; homelessness; inability to support the family; or incarceration. If a family's situation is severe, the infant and any other children may be removed and placed in foster care, with family treatment mandated as a component of the reunification process. Because of the requirement to report child abuse and neglect cases, the court and child protection services are often involved in mandated treatment. Itzkowitz (1989), Mansheim (1989), and Miller (1989) address such issues as families in the legal system, children in placement, and family violence.

Facilitating Parent–Infant Bonding

The first year of life is a critical period in the development of a parent–infant bond (Brazelton, 1972). The "dance of interaction" between a parent or caretaker and a child is essential for appropriate language, cognitive, intellectual, emotional, and social development. Many parents (particularly teenage or young parents) may not have a concrete idea of how this process happens. It is particularly important to coach young mothers and fathers on the bonding process during treatment sessions. Whenever possible, bonding should be encouraged and facilitated with young fathers as well as with mothers.

For a new parent, especially one with few supports, the basic "how-tos" of baby care can be very intimidating. A home-based family therapy session may be spent teaching (through modeling or coaching) a young parent how to bathe, hold, feed, quiet, burp, or change an infant. This facilitates bonding, because a parent who feels more in control or more competent is better able to enjoy the baby and to bond.

One of the most pleasurable exercises for a parent and child is infant massage. A parent can be taught to warm up his or her hands, use a baby lotion, and gently and lovingly massage the baby's body. The parent can be coached and encouraged to be playful (e.g., tickling and laughing with the baby) and to talk in soothing tones or sing a song to the infant.

Infants benefit from loving interactions with many family members. For example, helping a young grandmother (age 34) to teach her daughter (age 17) to bond with her baby will inevitably increase the bond among all three members of the family. It is important to keep in mind that other family members are there to support the parents and not to take over their role.

A clinician can work to schedule their home visits at a time when a baby's father (or the mother's boyfriend or the baby's grandfather) is home and can share in the experience. This can prove very challenging in the case of a teenage father. In many of these situations, the family of the teenage girl may be angry at the young man and unwilling to have him involved. A clinician may have to join first with the teenage girl and her extended family, and then gradually introduce the importance of father–child bonding. This can be a significant preventative intervention, which can have a major impact on the father's willingness to remain involved over the life of the child.

Bonding between the baby and other children in the household should not be forgotten. Siblings often feel abandoned when a new baby takes all of their mother's (and father's) attention. Involving them in these bonding sessions can help to minimize sibling rivalry. For example, after a mother has become quite adept at baby massage, she can coach her other child(ren) to participate in the process.

Groups can also be very helpful in facilitating bonding and child care education. The exercises mentioned above can be effective in a group of mothers, fathers, or parents who are all apprehensive. They can have the additional benefit of increasing the support and bonding between parents.

Case Example: Facilitating Bonding between a Homeless Teenage Mother and Her Newborn Son

Amy was a 16-year-old White adolescent referred by the hospital social worker after she gave birth prematurely to a son, Mark. Because of her pregnancy by her Black boyfriend, Amy had been thrown out of her home and placed in a foster home. Approximately 3 weeks prior to the birth, she moved in with her boyfriend and his mother. After an angry argument in which the boyfriend hit her, Amy went into labor and was rushed to the hospital by a neighbor. Both the boyfriend and his mother refused to have contact with her or the baby after this point.

Amy had a difficult labor and remained in the hospital for 1 week after giving birth. The family worker referred her to a transitional housing program at a residence for young mothers and their children.

Amy was terrified that she would not know how to care for her child. The worker coached Amy task by task in caring for her baby: holding, soothing, feeding, burping, and washing him. Most importantly, she fostered the bonding process. Amy and the worker also played together with Mark, with the worker encouraging their connection and bonding. With this attention, both Amy and her baby began to thrive.

PRESCHOOL CHILDREN

Unlike young children in prior decades, who were cared for at home until elementary school, the vast majority of children today attend some form of preschool, nursery, or day care program, or are cared for in someone else's home. Thus, the children's behavior and their families' parenting skills are observed by others when the children are still quite young. This means that preschool children are more frequently referred to early intervention programs than was formerly the case.

Children of this age are learning to speak with greater facility. Another major task at this time is the acquisition of social skills, including the ability to play and communicate with peers. As discussed above, families often need help with specific strategies for improving their parenting skills. A number of books and other resources give particularly helpful presentations of effective behavioral strategies for parents with young children. For example, *SOS: Help for Parents* (Clark, 1985a) is a well-illustrated, "parent-friendly" book that can be used directly with parents of young children. It gives clear strategies for handling "the terrible twos," the "no" stage, and acting out at home and in public (e.g., at supermarkets, in the car, etc.). The book also provides a number of excellent examples of "time-out" strategies and of positive reinforcers and appropriate punishments for young children. Finally, it helps parents to understand when they may be giving inconsistent messages. Clark (1985b) has also produced a video by the same name that can be used to train parents and therapists in these strategies. As the case of Billy (presented below) illustrates, these can be very effectively incorporated into a home-based family intervention. Problems in the home will frequently be manifested on the playground.

Case Example

Billy (age 4), a biracial child, and his African American mother, Latisha Ivey (age 28), were referred to a local family service agency by Billy's day care program. Billy had begun day care 6 months earlier and had initially been a very warm, friendly child who was well liked by other peers and teachers. Following his parents' separation 2 months prior to the referral, however, Billy became very angry. He hit other children in his preschool and often threw temper tantrums when asked by his teacher to do routine activities.

This intervention consisted of both home- and school-based components. (The school-based part of this intervention is described in Chapter 7.) The family worker had the initial meeting with Billy and Latisha in her office. It was apparent that Latisha was having a great deal of difficulty in controlling Billy. He told her "No!" and refused to sit in his seat when asked. When she tried to hold him on her lap, he hit her and broke free. Billy moved to a pile of toys in the corner of the office and began playing. The family worker used this opportunity to help Latisha talk about Billy's behavior and her own concerns. She reported that she and Billy's father had lived together for 4 years and had never married. Billy's father, George, was a White man (age 30) who had had a very stormy relationship with Latisha. In the few months prior to their separation, Latisha and George had had a number of angry arguments, which Billy often overheard. Finally, when George slapped her during an altercation, she told him to get out. She had not seen him since then, and he had had no contact with Billy.

Despite the problems in his parents' relationship, Latisha reported that Billy had enjoyed spending time with his father. They would often watch cartoons together, and Billy had loved to "cuddle" with his dad on Saturday mornings.

Billy was very direct in his anger at his mother. During the session he said to his mother. "You made Daddy go away." He then burst into tears. Latisha seemed at a loss as to what to do, and the therapist helped her to put her arms around her son and tell him that she loved him. This was difficult for Latisha, because she felt blamed by Billy and her entire family.

In the next session, the therapist agreed to come to the family's home because Latisha reported that Billy seemed out of control at home. It became clear that Billy's father had been the family disciplinarian and that Latisha had always deferred to him to manage Billy. George had often hit Billy when he misbehaved. Although Latisha did not "believe in hitting," she reported that she had gotten so "fed up" that she had spanked Billy a number of times. She began to cry and explained that she wished there was another way to make him behave. The therapist agreed that she would work with Latisha on changing her discipline strategies. The therapist also suggested family play therapy so that Billy could express his feelings in a nonthreatening way.

Family Play Therapy

The therapist had brought with her a medium-sized suitcase (which she kept in the trunk of her car), containing toys, crayons, paper, and other play materials. When she opened the suitcase in front of Billy, he became very interested in its contents. The therapist allowed him to pick out a toy he wanted to play with. He chose a baby dinosaur puppet. The therapist chose a slightly larger dinosaur puppet. Billy growled and yelled at the larger puppet. When the therapist asked who that puppet was, he said, "The daddy puppet." The therapist stated that the baby dinosaur was very angry at the daddy dinosaur. By now Billy was very engaged. The therapist played with him for about 15 minutes and then asked whether his mom would like to join them. Billy pulled another puppet out of the box and handed it to her. When the therapist asked Billy who this was, Billy said, "The mommy dinosaur."

The therapist, playing along, asked what the mommy dinosaur was doing. He said, "Crying." When asked why, he played out that she was mad at the daddy dinosaur and responded, "For leaving." Latisha, involved in the play, asked him what the mommy could have done. Billy replied, "Stop him from leaving" and "make him come back." The mother became defensive and started to explain herself. The therapist helped her to stay in the play and have the mommy dinosaur say to the baby, "I know you miss your daddy a lot and you wish that he could have stayed. I know you wish that I had a magic way to make him stay, but I could not." With the therapist supplying Latisha the words, she was able to share them with her son. The therapist encouraged her to have the mommy dinosaur hold the baby. Soon Billy and Latisha were embracing.

Parent Training

The next few sessions combined both behavioral parent training with the family play therapy. The worker helped Latisha to learn some basic parenting techniques so that she could feel more in control in her parenting of Billy. In the next session, when Billy again hit his mother, the therapist taught her how to hold him on her lap while holding his hands and telling him, "Hitting is not allowed." Billy calmed down and stopped struggling.

The therapist then began working with Latisha on the power of praise. When Billy chose a game from the therapist's collection and played it with his mother, the therapist modeled praise for Latisha and encouraged her to do likewise. Mother and son seemed closer when they left the session. In the next session, Latisha asked for help in thinking through handling acting-out behavior at home. The therapist discussed the value of time-out procedures with her, and Latisha agreed to try this procedure at home.

In the next session, Billy went straight to the puppets. He played with the three dinosaurs puppets for a few minutes, and then he had the mommy dinosaur say to the baby, "Hitting is not allowed. No hitting." With a big smile, he added, "Go to time out." He then giggled and danced around his mother and the therapist, obviously very pleased. The therapist and Latisha played this out under his direction a few more times.

In later sessions, the therapist helped Latisha to learn how to praise her son more systematically. She learned how to "catch him being good." In these sessions, she learned through modeling by the therapist and role playing how to praise her son for playing quietly while she and the therapist were talking.

The therapist also had a number of phone sessions with Billy's father, George, who refused to attend sessions in person. The parents were eventually able to work out a reasonable visitation and child support schedule. Billy saw his father every Saturday and began to thrive. His relationship with his mother continued to improve, as did his behavior in his preschool and at home.

Discussion

This example illustrates the power of play in family treatment with pre-school and school-age children. Eliana Gil (1994) has emphasized the importance of incorporating play into family therapy sessions. Unlike conventional play therapy, in which a therapist often works with a child separately, family members can be encouraged to share in the play scenarios. Artwork can also be very effective with preschool and school-age children and their families. A home-based family therapist can keep a "play corner" in a suitcase in the car, as the therapist in this case did. Materials such as puppets, dolls, toy soldiers, cars, blocks, and even a small dollhouse can be included, together with art supplies such as Magic Markers, crayons, paper, Play-Doh, and clay.

SCHOOL-AGE CHILDREN

Upon entering school, children encounter social and academic challenges that can cause difficulties for some. School-aged children may be referred for behavior problems such as oppositional defiant disorder, conduct disorder, or attention-deficit/hyperactivity disorder (ADHD), as well as symptoms of anxiety and depression. Clearly, the majority of referrals at this age are for "acting-out" children. Children who are very anxious, depressed, or withdrawn are frequently initially overlooked because they are not causing a problem for anyone. The following case illustrates the needs of these children and the ways in which home-based family treatment can address such issues.

Case Example

Melissa was an 8-year-old Puerto Rican child who was referred by her counselor at the parochial school she attended. She had been a very pleasant, well-behaved, and somewhat quiet child until the death of her father 6 months prior, after which she became very depressed and with-drawn. Her family consisted of her mother, Marta (age 34), and her brother, Felipe (age 7). Her family had left their small town in Puerto Rico 5 years previously in order to obtain better medical care for the father, Jorge, who had AIDS. The father's condition improved at first, but in the year prior to his death he had become more symptomatic and had lost weight rapidly. This was a very painful period in which the family had watched him "waste away and die."

Sister Roberta, the counselor at Melissa's school who referred the family, reported that the entire family seemed depressed and withdrawn. The therapist made an appointment to meet with the mother and the children at the school. It was clear that everyone was grieving for the death of the father. When the therapist asked whether the mother would prefer to have subsequent sessions in the clinic, the school, or the family's home, the mother responded that she would feel more comfortable meeting in her home, because "I don't come out much these days."

In the first home-based session, Marta sat on a couch, Melissa laid her head in her mother's lap, and Felipe sucked his thumb and rested his head on his mother's shoulder. Everyone looked profoundly depressed. The therapist stated that they all seemed very sad. Melissa began to cry, and before long her mother and brother were also in tears. Marta embraced her children, and the therapist had the sense of a family that was extremely close; Marta reinforced this when she described them as "joined at the hip."

Marta talked about how hard they had prayed for a "miracle" to cure the father. When the father was first treated in the United States, the combination of medication was effective, and the father seemed stronger. The "miracle" they had sought from praying to St. Jude (the patron of hopeless causes) and the Virgin Mary appeared to have happened. But after 4 years, when the treatments lost their effectiveness and the father's condition began to decline, Marta stated that they "all went downhill" and "everyone became very sad." Jorge spent increasingly large blocks of time in the hospital and was "totally out of it" when he was at home, sleeping most of the time.

Marta reported that both children had been very close to their father. Melissa was his "princess" and Felipe was his "prince." The therapist asked each of the children about their memory of their father and his nicknames for them. Both children became more engaged during the session. Melissa reported, "Yes, he always called me his princess. I loved him a lot." Felipe responded, "I miss him a lot." The session ended with Marta agreeing to another home-based session a week later.

In the next session, Marta reported that during the week Felipe had been repeatedly asking, "Where has Daddy gone?" and "When is he coming back?" The therapist took some colored markers and three sheets of paper out of her suitcase of play materials, and asked each member of the family to draw a picture of where they thought their Dad had gone. They each drew their version of "heaven." Felipe had a picture of a grave and a little stick figure of a boy crying. Melissa drew a picture of heaven with winged angels flying. Marta drew a grave and a few clouds. When the family members were asked to share stories about their pictures, Felipe cried and reported that he didn't know where his father was. The therapist encouraged Marta to hold Melissa and Felipe, and to tell them what her beliefs were about their father's death and "where he is now."

Marta shared her Catholic religious belief that Jorge had gone home to God and was in heaven and was happy and at peace. Melissa showed Felipe her pictures of angels and told him that the angels would take care of their father. Felipe asked again, "But when is he coming back?" Marta again became tearful and hugged him. The therapist sat close to Marta and Felipe and said in a quiet voice, "I know you miss your daddy so much and want him to come back, but he won't be coming back. He will be waiting for you in heaven." Marta, taking her cue from the therapist, held Felipe and Melissa and told them that some day they would see him again in heaven.

In subsequent sessions, artwork was frequently incorporated into family sessions and seemed to be a very helpful vehicle in allowing all family members to express their feelings.

In one session, the therapist asked all family members to work together on a large piece of paper and draw their "best memories" of their dad. All three members of the family became very engaged. Marta drew him walking out of the hospital looking well, as he had after first receiving treatment in the United States. Felipe drew a picture of his father playing ball with him back home in Puerto Rico when he was very little. Melissa drew a picture of a very tall man (her dad) carrying a tiny girl (herself) on his shoulders. This was a particularly moving session.

In one session about 2 months later, they each drew a picture of the family without their father. Melissa drew a large, empty hole with three small pebbles. Felipe drew three tiny stick figures at the bottom of a large sheet of paper. Marta drew three people in a boat with high waves washing over it. She said, "They are adrift at sea." The mourning process continued over many months.

One week, a very anxious Marta greeted the family worker as she entered the house with the news that the father's birthday would have been next week. This became the topic of the session. With the therapist's help, they talked about prior birthday celebrations in which the whole family went out to dinner. Marta stated that she had been thinking of visiting his grave to place flowers, but she was torn about taking the children. The therapist encouraged her to ask each of the children what they thought about this. Melissa responded immediately that she wanted to go and leave flowers too. Felipe, very hesitantly, stated that he wanted to go but was "scared." The therapist asked what he was scared of. He reported that he had seen a TV movie about haunted graveyards. His mother was able to reassure him that his father's graveyard was not haunted. The therapist suggested that the family visit the grave as planned and then go out to dinner together afterward.

In the next session, everyone appeared relaxed and far less sad and depressed than in previous weeks. The therapist helped to connect Marta with a support group for people whose spouses had died, and to connect the children with a support group for children who had lost a parent. Both groups were run by a local hospice program.

Within the following year, the whole family had shown improvement. The children were engaging more with their friends at school, and Marta had become friendly with a woman in the support group who had also lost her husband. Anniversaries such as Father's Day, family members' birthdays, and holidays such as Thanksgiving, and Christmas were still very difficult, but gradually each family member was able to go on with life.

Discussion

This case illustrates the power of home-based outreach. Initially, Marta and the children had all withdrawn from the outside world. The home-based intervention met them where they were, and the therapist then gradually worked to connect them with outside supports and peers, through the support groups run by the hospice program.

This case also illustrates the value of family artwork (Gil, 1994) in home-based family treatment. This provided a vehicle for the family members to express their grief and share it with each other.

SUMMARY

As children are being referred at earlier and earlier ages, family workers must be prepared with intervention strategies appropriate for young children and their families. Reaching out to family members in their homes, providing multisystems support, and using vehicles such as toys and drawing materials so that family members can more comfortably express painful issues will enable these families to provide an environment in which at-risk children may flourish.

Therapists can make a major contribution by providing education about appropriate parenting practices at different ages. They can find creative ways to utilize the families' strengths, including extended family and friend resources, to make the tasks of parenting less burdensome. Parents and family members who feel nourished and praised by their therapists will be more capable of nurturing and positively reinforcing their children's behavior. Parents who, in addition, are connected with others through support groups will feel less isolated and will have these networks available long after the treatment ends (see Chapter 8).

CHAPTER 6

Working with Adolescents and Their Families

This chapter describes how to incorporate behavioral (Falloon, 1991) and social learning principles (Patterson & Forgatch, 1987) into home-based family therapy work with adolescents and their families. It should be noted here that most of our interventions with adolescents also involve individual school-based sessions and work with the school staff. This chapter focuses on individual work with adolescents and family therapy in their homes. The school-based interventions are discussed in Chapter 7.

UNDERSTANDING WHAT MOTIVATES BEHAVIOR

Practitioners need working assumptions about the causes of individuals' day-to-day, moment-to-moment functioning. Then, they will know what to target if they wish to influence that functioning. We have found, for instance, that it is useful to view adolescent development as a dynamic process. Adolescents are changing and developing every day. They are constantly learning through trial and error. They are continually experimenting with new ways to cope and "ways to be," and adopting or rejecting these behaviors and views of themselves for the future.

The underlying assumption of this dynamic view is that human behavior is learned and pragmatic, and is thus changeable (Biglan, 1995). It is shaped by moment-to-moment interactions with its context. Adolescents essentially do what pays off—in the short run—for them. If they do their homework, but find that the activity has not paid off, they are less likely to do it in the future. If they tease a friend in the classroom, and it pays off with an immediate smile or laugh, they are more likely to do it in the future. "Payoff" is individually determined; what is rewarding for one adolescent may be punishing for another.

According to social learning theory, adolescents learn what to do from what happens *after* they do it—from feedback or the results of the action. In order to influence the adolescents' direction, therapists want to give as much feedback as possible. Understanding that adolescents learn to do things as a function of both accidental and expected consequences enables practitioners to intervene judiciously to influence what adolescents do. Wherever possible, workers should try to ensure that adolescents receive immediate payoffs for positive behavior and not for negative behavior.

Because therapists are often not there when positive behavior occurs, they must coordinate efforts with the other adults in the adolescents' environment. Once a therapist identifies or assesses what an adolescent must do to "go in the right direction," the therapist (1) lets the adolescent know that he or she notices whenever the adolescent takes even the smallest steps in the right direction; (2) talks to teachers, coaches, and probation officers about acknowledging those steps too; and (3) coordinates with family members so that they can acknowledge them as well. (See Bry & Krinsley, 1990, for the application of these principles to an adolescent case.)

ENGAGING WITH ADOLESCENTS AND THEIR FAMILIES

It is vital to connect with an adolescent individually, in addition to working with the parents. This can be done by having individual sessions with the adolescent in addition to those with the entire family, or by dividing a single session into two or three components.

For work with an adolescent, the therapist should take responsibility for providing an experience that the adolescent will want to repeat (or at least not mind repeating). It is not helpful for a therapist to attribute an unsuccessful session to characteristics of the client. Circumstances that make the adolescent uncomfortable, such as not giving the adolescent sufficient "space" (e.g., looking directly across a small table) or asking questions too difficult to answer, should be avoided. If the therapist cannot find a way to change these uncomfortable conditions, the negative aspects of intervention may override the positive ones, causing the adolescent to refuse to continue meeting.

The therapist should avoid assigning blame to the adolescent. For example, rather than saying, "Your poor grades made this necessary," or "I am here because of your suspensions from school," the proactive practitioner communicates, "I want to work with you," "I want to see you graduate," "I want you to get to class on time," and "I want to see you next week." Note that the practitioner does not risk asking the adolescent whether he or she wants to continue working together. (Very few adolescents are eager for therapy.)

It is optimal to plan individual sessions with adolescents at sites where they will be in the course of the day (i.e., at home or at school), and at times that are convenient to them. The more convenient the sessions are for the adolescents, the more likely they are to participate.

Having empathy and respect for an adolescent and family is as important as having a proactive stance and an understanding of what motivates them. It is far more effective to operate from the assumption that all family members are coping in the best way they know how with their life circumstances than to think in terms of intractable psychopathology, personality traits, or dysfunctions. Because the therapist, teachers, and family all want the same thing—for the adolescent to grow up and be able to support himself or herself independently as an adult—they each will be more powerful and effective if they work together instead of judging each other. Our approach is entirely consistent with solution-focused therapy in this regard (Berg, 1994).

Therapists are advised to use a variation on the Golden Rule as a guide to reaching out: "Let us do with parents (and teachers) only what we would want someone to do with us." We need to recognize that parents are busy with their own lives. As previously discussed, some parents, particularly low-income parents who have had to apply for financial assistance or deal with child protective services, have experienced outside agencies as making their lives harder. When we realize how strange and difficult it would be for us to meet with an outsider who came to our house to talk about our children, we can be more patient and understanding when we have to reschedule meetings multiple times.

BEHAVIORAL ASSESSMENT

Assessment for an outreach worker involves an adolescent and those in the adolescent's environment—peers, the neighborhood, the family, and the school. First, the therapist should consider the reasons for the referral and the expectations of the family and the adolescent. Adolescents may be referred for a range of problems, including ADHD, eating disorders, learning difficulties, juvenile delinquency and court involvement, conduct disorder, or depression. Because many of the young people family therapists see come to them through prevention projects, they also assess "at-risk" adolescents. With such a youth, a therapist should be particularly aware of any measurable "warning signs" that would concern most objective people, such as poor school attendance, failing grades in courses, suspensions from school, and arrests by the police. After gaining permission, the therapist should obtain any relevant documents, such as school attendance records, report cards, discipline records, or arrest records (see Chapter 7).

Interviewing the Adolescent and Family

Assessment should always include an individual interview with the adolescent (or a session can be divided, giving the adolescent and the parent(s) each time alone and a time when they are all together). The therapist should elicit the youth's views on the presenting problem and learn as much as possible about the daily surrounding circumstances of the adolescent, including names and relationships of family members and friends. (Bry, Greene, Schutte, & Fishman's [1991] *Targeted Family Intervention Manual* covers the most important specific areas to assess.)

An essential step of our approach is to learn about a "dream" that an adolescent carries around. A "dream" is something that the adolescent would like to do or have in 5 or 10 years. It is sometimes difficult for an adolescent to express a dream, so it may be helpful for the therapist to guess if the adolescent says he or she cannot think of anything. Common "dreams" are to be a rap star, a basketball or football player, a secretary, or a Lexus owner; to have a house, spouse, and children; to have one's own business, such as an electrical repair shop; or to work as a disc jockey or the mixer for a musical group. Once the adolescent shares a dream, the therapist accepts it as it is; he or she does not alter it or evaluate with the adolescent how realistic it is. Instead, the therapist keeps it in reserve, to introduce gently into a conversation when motivation flags or the relevance of a difficult task eludes the adolescent.

The first stage of assessment ends with interviews with members of the adolescent's family and a visit to the neighborhood. Their views on the presenting problem and on family strengths are elicited. Daily circumstances are discussed. For example, in the face of chronic tardiness, the family is asked about the method by which the adolescent is awakened, what means of transportation is used to get to school, and so on. It is useful to draw a genogram, including family members *and* friends. Finally, any further problems that specifically concern the parents are collected, such as fighting with siblings, staying out all night without telling them, or coming home high.

Conceptualizing the Situation

Consistent with a learning formulation, the therapist conceptualizes the adolescent's and family's situation in terms of specific, discrete behaviors and thoughts. For example, in a family where an adolescent has a habit of yelling out insulting things to teachers in class, and a mother has a habit of thinking that she has too many problems of her own to worry about her child's, a behavioral family therapist will operate from the assumption that the adolescent and mother have learned to behave and think this way and that they are able to learn to behave and think a different way instead. This is a hopeful, optimistic formulation, in contrast to the more prevalent pessimistic formulation in terms of personality characteristics and dispositions (i.e., characterizing the adolescent as "an angry kid" and the mother as "a rejecting mother," which sounds less changeable and more pathological). Dattilio (1998) presents a case in which parents and their adolescent improved their relationship by learning to think differently.

Next the therapist assesses exactly what actions and thoughts increase the adolescent's negative behaviors or risk factors. In other words, the next step in a behavioral assessment is to determine why the adolescent and the mother behave and think in the way that they do. Under what circumstances did they learn these behaviors and thoughts? What "payoffs" are there for their continuing to do it? What stops them from behaving and thinking differently? Such an assessment is often called a "functional analysis" (Robin & Foster, 1989).

Family therapists find out the answers to these questions by asking for details about one instance of problem behavior or thinking at a time. To find out how the actions or thoughts benefit each person, therapists should ascertain what happens immediately afterward. Actions and thoughts that may appear self-defeating to outsiders may have an immediate, positive payoff for an individual. For instance, instead of doing homework, an adolescent may watch television or talk to friends on the phone. The disapproval that the adolescent experiences from the teacher the next day or at the end of the grading period is hours or weeks removed from the time during which he or she would have done homework. Likewise, the immediate result of a mother's thinking that her teenage son is old enough to take care of himself is the avoidance of a terrible feeling of helplessness if she were instead to think it was *her* responsibility to keep him from, for instance, "joyriding" in stolen cars with his friends.

Goal Setting

The final stage of assessment is the development of intervention goals. This is often harder to do well than it looks. First, the therapist must package all of the multiple problems into four to six discrete, achievable outcomes of the intervention whose relevance is clear to the adolescent and parents. Second, as suggested above, the goals should be stated in positive, observable terms (i.e., in terms of what the improvement will look like). If all one has heard is a stream of negative complaints from the adolescent and/or parents, formulating this list is challenging. Berg (1994) provides helpful guidance on goal setting. It is useful to target very specific observable behaviors—for example, school attendance or school performance. The list of goals for the adolescent can include some items that are not shared with the parents, such as "Save money for a moped by buying marijuana less often," and the goals for the parents can include items that the adolescent doesn't value, such as "Know where my daughter is when she goes out."

The outcome goals are written down by the therapist, revised (if necessary) with input from the adolescent and parents, and then agreed to by all concerned. These goals guide the intervention. Despite crises and other issues that inevitably arise from week to week, the therapist endeavors to ask each week about evidence of goal attainment: "What grades did you get in Mrs. Jackson's class this week?", "How many days did you manage to stay in class and out of the discipline room?", or "Did you get Mary's birth certificate for her working papers?" Therapist, adolescent, and family members alike will appreciate that the intervention is "targeted" in this way.

Once the goals are set, the next challenge is facilitating the adolescent's progress toward the specified outcomes. A therapist should use the following standard as a guide for each activity: Will this activity increase the probability of meeting the targeted goals? That is, will this activity lead to greater payoff for targeted positive behavior or decreased payoff for assessed negative behavior? And will this activity increase protective factors in the adolescent's life or decrease risk factors? (See Chapter 10 for a discussion of protective and risk factors.)

Before seeing the adolescent and family members each week, the therapist should try to ascertain from independent sources, such as the school or probation officer, what the adolescent has done in the past week regarding his or her goals. The therapist should also establish what the adolescent must do in the following week in order to continue to stay out of trouble. These nontraditional aspects of the intervention help the practitioner to prevent someone from inadvertently rewarding problem behavior (e.g., by offering praise or a special shopping trip) on the basis of incomplete information. Additional information also enables the practitioner to use sessions more productively, as the adolescent will frequently say that "everything is okay" or that "nothing happened" when asked what happened in the previous week. Of course, the therapist should be sure to have the correct release forms from the adolescent and family before approaching independent sources for information (see the discussion of confidentiality in Chapter 7).

In weekly sessions with the adolescent and/or with the adolescent and family, the therapist tries to ascertain what payoffs may be maintaining the adolescent's problematic behavior and what payoffs can be arranged when the adolescent takes steps toward the intervention goals. Examples of payoffs include the following: The therapist may praise homework completion; the therapist and a parental figure may agree that the adolescent will receive an allowance if he or she does a chore, such as taking out the garbage or cooking a meal; the therapist may help the adolescent get a new privilege or freedom at home, at school, or in the community; and so on. Sometimes, by merely monitoring whether or not preexisting plans have been carried out, the therapist can add crucial acknowledgment for a lot of little extra efforts on the adolescent's and family's parts. These strategies do not differ greatly from individual or family therapy sessions in a clinic. The nontraditional aspects are that they occur in an adolescent's home or school.

Eventually, therapists "work themselves out of jobs" by arranging for the payoffs for good adolescents' behavior to occur without their presence. This may take anywhere from a few months to a few years, if necessary. Even then, therapists should arrange increasingly infrequent booster sessions with adolescents and families (Bry & Krinsley, 1992). If a crisis arises, however, a therapist will of course become more active again for such time as is necessary. And all along, weekly indicators concerning the goals, such as school attendance, are monitored for either improvement or backsliding.

SPECIFIC INTERVENTION STRATEGIES

Positive Feedback

The first change that family therapists effect in adolescents' environments is the presence of the therapists themselves. Werner (1989) found in her longitudinal study of Kauai children with risk factors that a positive outcome was generally associated with the presence of a surrogate parent in a child's life—an interested adult or a teacher. It should be noted that a practitioner does not compete with or supplant the parent or family, but adds to, extends, and supplements parenting.

As Chapter 10 documents, consistent, positive parenting promotes a more problem-free adolescence. The presence of a therapist in an adolescent's life increases positive parenting in two ways: The therapist both reinforces the positive parenting of the parents or guardians and influences the adolescent directly through positive feedback. The therapist knows that he or she is exerting a positive influence when the adolescent voluntarily reports accomplishing something that the therapist values, such as "Guess what! I got an A on the math quiz today!" or "John kicked my books today, and I wasn't sent to the vice-principal because I didn't kick his books back."

Therapists respond differently to what adolescents say than do their friends, teachers, parents, and family members. Sternberg and Bry (1994) demonstrated the impact of therapists' reactions. In sessions where therapists acknowledged new ideas by saying, "That's an idea," clients generated more new ideas than they did in sessions where these were not specifically acknowledged.

Practitioners will also find many "teaching moments" with adolescents—times when they can prompt appropriate behavior naturally, and times when they can shape new behavior by ignoring actions that are less effective and responding to those that are more effective. For example, when a combative adolescent sulks and appears not to like what is happening in a session, the therapist can prompt the adolescent to state a preference about the session *and can respond positively to the verbalized preference*, thus teaching the adolescent that verbalizing can be an effective method to get needs met.

In family sessions, parents often need prompting to acknowledge the good behavior that does occur, even though they wish there were more of it. Going over an adolescent's report card subject by subject with the parents and adolescent together and pointing out where grades have gone up, where teachers' comments have improved, and where absences have gone down is a very effective intervention strategy.

Some parents state that they do not believe in praising children for "things they should be doing anyway." Then the therapist can reframe what they are doing as "telling Tyrone what things he's done that are the kind of things that we like to see—to make sure that he knows what we think." Each intervention needs to be suited to the individual adolescent and family. When one mother could not be persuaded to try to influence her son's activities directly because they were "in God's hands," the therapist was able to persuade her to pray out loud in her son's presence so that he could hear what she was praying for.

Given the amount of short-term benefits that there are for negative behavior, it is not surprising that adolescents persist in doing things that defeat themselves in the long run (Gottfredson & Hirschi, 1994). The basis for the interventions we describe is the assumption that if therapists can increase the short-term benefits for positive behavior, adolescents will spend more time engaging in such behavior. And the more often they repeat positive behavior and experience benefits for it, the more likely it is to become well-learned behavior in the future.

Being a Role Model

The therapist is also an important role model for both adolescents and parents, representing—at the most basic level—someone who has graduated from school and has gotten and kept a good job. There are additional ways in which the therapist teaches by example. One key area is obeying rules. For example, the therapist should always model asking permission from parents if he or she plans to see an adolescent after school, or to keep the adolescent late.

Although therapists do not perform a disciplinary role, they can point out the penalties that are usually associated with specific adolescent actions. For example, a therapist can say to an adolescent, "Make sure to turn in this homework we've worked on together, because just a few zeroes for homework can pull a grade point average into the F range," "A person who drives a car without a license in this state, loses the chance to get a license for 2 years," "Just being in the same car or in the same room with someone who has drugs means you can be convicted of possession," or "Yes, the principal has the right to suspend you for a week. The school handbook says that's the penalty for what you did." Adolescents' awareness of the penalties for problem behavior has been found to be a powerful protective factor (Stephens, 1996).

The family therapist can also model delaying gratification. Clients will notice a therapist driving a modestly priced car instead of the Lexus that they dream about, or wearing the same business-like outfit during several meetings instead of having an extensive wardrobe of designer clothes.

Finally, the therapist can also demonstrate life management skills—for instance, "I'm leaving right after our session today because I have a meeting with my supervisor, and I want to allow extra time in case I'm caught in traffic."

Monitoring

Another protective factor that the therapist can provide is monitoring an adolescent's activities—both by keeping the adolescent's parents or guardians informed about the adolescent's life outside the home, and by monitoring the adolescent's activities himself or herself. Just knowing that adults are aware of what they are doing has a powerful positive effect on adolescents' behavior. Beier (1990) found that even adolescents who used drugs an average of 5 days a week chose not to use drugs on days when they feared their parents would find out. It is our experience that the same applies to the adolescent–therapist relationship; that is, an adolescent is more likely to do the right thing if he or she thinks that the therapist will find out.

Outside of school (see Chapter 7), the monitoring that has the greatest impact on adolescent outcomes is parents' knowledge about where their children are when they are not home (Stice, Myers, & Brown, 1998). In addition to keeping parents informed about what their children are doing in school, the most important thing that therapists can do is to encourage parents repeatedly to ask their adolescents to tell them where they are going whenever they are not home. Therapists might want to discuss with both parents and children methods for facilitating this communication (e.g., keeping a pad next to the telephone, purchasing an answering machine or voice mail system, supplying a sufficient quantity of quarters so that adolescents may use public telephones at any time). If a therapist can only make this one change in the home life of an adolescent, it may be enough, in and of itself, to prevent negative outcomes.

Increasing Adult Involvement

Another protective factor against adolescent problems is actual involvement by adults in the lives of adolescents (Krohn & Thornberry, 1993). This can include therapists' and parents' talking to the adolescents' friends, going to school open houses, watching them play sports, attending science fairs, and helping them to get and keep jobs (Rigsby, Stull, & Morse-Kelley, 1997). Involvement also means taking an interest in all of the life details that are important to an adolescent but may have little or nothing to do with the goals of the intervention, such as remembering the adolescent's boyfriend's or girlfriend's name, as well as learning his or her preferences in music, clothes, jewelry, sports, TV shows, and movies. Not only does this involvement communicate interest in the adolescent as a person, but regular discussions about these issues can enhance the adolescent's sense of choice and control over life.

When sufficient trust has been developed, the adolescent may acknowledge realities to the therapist that he or she has found too difficult to acknowledge before.

For instance, one adolescent stopped going to practice for the high school basketball team, even though he was a talented and sought-after player. He told his friends and mother that he'd stopped playing because he was not interested in basketball any more and because the coach was a "jerk." His therapist, however, who had seen him play and who knew the coach, was able to help him articulate that he had dropped out because he could not read or remember the plays. This recognition motivated the adolescent to accept a placement in a school for students with learning disabilities. Meanwhile, he resumed playing "pickup" basketball in his neighborhood.

Engaging in Advocacy

Because therapists work with so many adolescents, they know more than most parents can know about what opportunities are available for adolescents and how youth-oriented social systems work (Boyd-Franklin, 1989; Henggeler et al., 1998). They can inform adolescents, parents, and other family members about opportunities, guide them through the application process, and call up program directors to make sure that their applications will be considered.

Adults can advocate for adolescents in several ways: by influencing salient adults' impressions, by drawing attention to otherwise overlooked adolescents, and by convincing the adolescents themselves that they are good enough to take advantage of opportunities available to them. Therapists can be instrumental in obtaining subsidized lunches for eligible students. They can help get students who have shown an interest in or proficiency for the subject matter to enroll in vocational high schools. They may be instrumental in facilitating students' entries into recreational sports, such as cheerleading, intramural basketball, and summer football practice. Therapists are also aware of summer job programs for low-income adolescents. Getting into one of these programs can change the trajectory of a youth's life. Publicity about these programs does not get to the majority of parents, particularly those who are highly stressed or those who have several children with problems (Parece, 1997). In addition, the application process is unusually demanding and requires multiple steps. Without the advocacy of family workers, many opportunities for adolescents do not come to the notice of adolescents and their parents, or parents unknowingly fail to complete the entire application process and remain ignorant as to why their adolescents did not get into the program. One word of caution is indicated here. As advocated in Chapter 3, it is very important that family workers not "take over" the job of the parents but, rather, empower them to do this advocacy on their own behalf.

Advocacy can also make a substantial difference in ensuring constructive intervention. A therapist who tells a judge in the juvenile justice system that an adolescent and family have been attending counseling weekly and using the time well can increase the possibility that the adolescent is sentenced to a term of house arrest or probation instead of incarceration.

Although much of workers' advocacy will occur *on behalf* of adolescents, they may also advocate directly *to* adolescents and parents. For example, extracurricular activities for an adolescent can complicate a parent's life. The parent may be concerned about extra expenses, about demands for transportation, about the adolescent's being with people whom the parent does not know and trust, and about the adolescent's unavailability for the parent. Likewise, adolescents may be conflicted about participating in extracurricular activities. They may feel inadequate or unconfident; they may be afraid of rejection or uncomfortable in strange company; or they may feel powerless in a setting where they do not know how things work.

Adolescents and parents may express criticism of programs or they may simply remain inactive, but fear is probably behind their objections. Respectful inquiring will often lead to hints about these fears. For example, a parent might say, "I don't have that kind of money," or an adolescent might say, "I can't run for Student Council because I've had detention." Each fear can be anticipated, assessed, and addressed. The therapist should discuss the facts and correct any misconceptions. For example, he or she can say to the parent, "Scholarships are available, and I know several parents have applied because they want their children to have this opportunity." Or the therapist can say to the adolescent, "I'll bet there are other Student Council members who get into trouble sometimes. I know I did when I was on Student Council."

Parents should be encouraged to advocate for their children. When parents are involved in the selection of their children's friends, this serves as a protective factor against early drug use (Catalano et al., 1992). Adolescents whose parents actively help them get jobs, instead of letting them fend for themselves, enjoy their work more, which suggests that they will keep their jobs longer (Cotton & Bynum, 1995).

Teaching Problem Solving and Communication

A significant skill for adolescents and their families to learn is step-by-step problem solving. This consists of (1) identifying a problem (from the standpoint of the person who feels the most concerned), (2) generating alternative solutions, (3) selecting the least problematic one, (4) planning implementation, and (5) reevaluating the plan according to the outcome (D'Zurilla, 1986; Robin & Foster, 1989; Sanders & Dadds, 1993). In a multiproblem family, a therapist may never get past the first step— identifying the problem. It can sometimes take an entire family session to formulate one discrete problem and decide who "owns" it. Even if the therapist does not help the family with the other problem-solving steps, he or she can nevertheless stimulate tremendous positive change by merely helping to identify just one discrete problem.

It is not easy to identify a problem. This process involves not only selecting one discrete problem out of many, but also describing it in viewable terms, clarifying for whom it is a problem (this is often not the person the family may have originally selected), and deciding why it is a problem for that person (i.e., what emotional difference it makes to him or her).

It is important that the therapist keep asking the family to delay discussing possible solutions to the problem until the identification process described above is completed. If family members do not hold off on considering solutions, they could go through an unnecessary and possibly destructive discussion of a misidentified problem. For instance, they might try to solve a misidentified problem ("Jamie's obsession with boys") instead of the real problem ("Mother's loneliness when Jamie is out Saturday nights").

Ideally, the family member who is most upset by a problem will present it in the form of an "I statement." An "I statement" begins with the words "I feel . . ." and continues immediately with a word describing a vulnerable emotion. Examples are "I feel afraid," "I feel hopeless," "I feel disappointed," or "I feel misunderstood."

Most therapists who guide families and couples through problem solving have found that they must do "I statement" communication training first (Blechman, 1985; Bry & Krinsley, 1990; Jacobson, 1984; McCrady & Epstein, 1995; Robin & Foster, 1989). Therapists function as directors, actively coaching family members how to talk to each other without accusations and how to listen to each other without interruptions. No specific time in therapy sessions is designated for communication training. Instead, family members are promptly coached to make "I statements" whenever blaming statements occur in the course of conversation.

It is essential for a practitioner to keep up communication training throughout therapy. Genuine "I statements" drastically reduce arguments (which can lead families to discontinue family sessions) because the therapist can remind family members that such statements merely describe one person's subjective reaction and that others will have different, albeit equally valid, reactions to the same situation. The therapist actively interrupts arguing by saying that no one needs to defend himself or herself because no one is being blamed.

During communication training, a therapist must be careful not to stop the "I statement" formation process too early (i.e., when the person who is most concerned has identified only judgment or anger instead of a vulnerable emotion). Many people will unknowingly disguise blame by saying "I feel that . . ." when they really mean "I think." Then they end up stating a negative opinion or judgment about someone else, which can lead to an argument, instead of a subjective reaction, which is about only themselves.

An effective question to help clients discover their emotions about a problem is "What difference does it make to you?" or "What does it mean to you?" Even after a client answers these questions, however, a therapist usually has to guess (respectfully) what vulnerable emotion the problem generates until the right word is found. Skilled therapists, therefore, must have an extensive vocabulary of "feeling words" at their disposal so that they can find the precise ones that clients will accept. Lindblad-Goldberg, Dore, and Stern (1998) actually teach families how to make "I feel . . ." statements before they begin their very first in-home sessions.

For instance, to an adolescent who says, "The problem is that Mrs. Harris didn't give us enough time to read our books before the report was due," a therapist may respond, "So you're worried that your report won't be done on time?" The adolescent may not accept the word "afraid," but may accept the word "worried." Another example is a parent who complains, "The problem is that Jennifer can't tell time." After much exploration about who "owns" the problem (the parent) and what the problem means emotionally to the parent, the therapist may help the parent say, "When Jennifer is not home by her curfew, I feel scared that she is dead." The therapist helps the family change the focus of the problem from blaming another person to the vulnerable emotions of the person who is most concerned about the problem.

With some families and adolescents, we have learned to avoid the word "problem," for they do not want to see themselves as having problems. We use the words "concern," "worry," "fear," "issue," or "challenge" instead. A motivational strategy that we strenuously avoid—one that many teachers and parents use habitually—is trying to prove to adolescents and parents that they have problems or that they are wrong. We do not use the confrontation strategy of some substance abuse treatment programs. We do not take away clients' self-esteem. The reason is that clients can more easily take action to better their lives from a position of feeling good about themselves than from one of feeling bad about themselves.

Besides helping adolescents and parents define discrete concerns from the emotional standpoint of the speaker, therapists also help them address just one problem at a time. When other problems are mentioned, a therapist can respectfully say, "Let's first finish discussing your disappointment over finding dirty dishes in the sink when you get home from work. Then we can later discuss your concern about food being left in the bedrooms." For some families, the habit of addressing just one problem at a time is the most useful skill that they learn from their practitioners.

Targeting Beliefs

Yet another intervention strategy involves targeting and changing beliefs or assumptions that can impede positive action (Dattilio, 1998; Robin & Foster, 1989). As a preliminary step, clients must learn how to identify and examine their beliefs. Practitioners encourage such a focus by paraphrasing the thoughts that adolescents and parents mention as they recount events. The types of thoughts that therapists consider targeting for change are explanatory statements, causal explanations, characterizations of people in order to explain their reactions, attributions of cause, and statements about how the world works. Examples that we have heard from adolescents and parents include the following: "That principal hates all of my kids," "Mr. Bennett favors girls," "I can't do math," "I'll never be able to learn Spanish," "The police are out to get him," "College is corny," "Only dorks work on the school newspaper," "I have turned him over to the Lord and washed my hands of responsibility for him," "It's his father's responsibility [who lives in the next town] to raise my son [who lives in her house]," "Drugs don't affect me," "He's not my friend because he does not phone me," "I don't need to hand in my makeup work because the teacher did not ask me for it," "Summer camp costs too much," "I can't apply for a job because my mother can't find my birth certificate," "My daughter wants to flunk out of school," and "My child is trying to upset me."

We consistently find that families and adolescents with problems explain events in more pessimistic ways, with greater learned helplessness, and with less of a future orientation (Parker, 1995; Seligman, 1990; Stephens, 1996; Turk, 1993; Turk & Bry, 1992). Their explanations for negative events tend to be personalized, pervasive, and permanent; their explanations for positive events tend to be more external to themselves, more temporary, and specific only to the event being explained.

Hearing clients give pessimistic causal explanations, however, should not make therapists pessimistic. As mentioned earlier, therapists should assume that clients came to think this way through learning processes and thus can come to think differently likewise through learning processes. The methods a therapist can use to change a client's thinking are as follows: (1) identifying the explanatory belief through paraphrasing it as a belief instead of as a fact; (2) respectfully asking the speaker to reexamine the stated belief by paraphrasing it with a questioning tone; (3) reinforcing a possible alternative explanation if the client offers one; (4) offering palatable (to the client and to the therapist) alternative explanations if the client does not offer one; (5) disconnecting the belief from the client's response if the client rejects the alternative explanations; and (6) trying to find or arrange a corrective experience, in which the counselor can point to an alternative cause for the event that the adolescent and parent will accept.

An example of such an interchange during a home-based session follows:

ADOLESCENT: Mrs. Smith isn't fair. She gave me an F just because I didn't hand in *one* homework!

THERAPIST: You think just *one* zero pulled your grade all the way down to an F? [Paraphrasing adolescent's thought as a belief instead of as a fact and asking her to reexamine it])

GRANDMOTHER: That teacher's always picking on my Jasmine.

ADOLESCENT: She *said* I got the F because of that one homework.

THERAPIST: Well, I know that the principal has been telling the teachers to get tough, and the principal's Mrs. Smith's boss. Perhaps Mrs. Smith had no choice. [Offering an alternative explanation.]

ADOLESCENT: She didn't give other kids an F for missing just one homework.

GRANDMOTHER: Can she do that?

THERAPIST: Well, teachers *can* decide what homework they're going to count in the grade and what homework they're not going to count in the grade. So, Jasmine, if you hand in every single homework that's due this next grading period, Mrs. Smith won't be *able* to give you an F. You'll keep her from being unfair. [Disconnecting the belief from client's response.]

ADOLESCENT: Whatever.

THERAPIST (*to both Jasmine and Grandmother*): There are teacher–parent conferences next Tuesday night. I'd like to meet with Mrs. Smith and see what she says about this. Do you want to come with me? [Trying to arrange a corrective experience.]

GRANDMOTHER: No, you know I never go out at night.

THERAPIST: I'll tell you what. I'll meet you here at 7:00 P.M. Tuesday, and we can go over together. How's that?

GRANDMOTHER: Okay. We'll go together.

JASMINE: I want to go too.

THERAPIST (to Grandmother): Is that okay with you?

GRANDMOTHER: Yes.

THERAPIST: Okay. I'll meet you both here at 7:00 on Tuesday. I'll call before I come.

Although therapists do not necessarily expect adolescents to develop empathy for teachers (or parents), they can nevertheless offer, as alternative explanations, reframes that portray authority figures as people who have their own vulnerabilities. Despite the fact that such alternative explanations may be rejected when they are offered, therapists are sometimes rewarded weeks later by hearing their words used by adolescents or parents to explain a new event. One-trial learning, however, seldom occurs. Instead, a therapist usually must offer an alternative explanation and point out evidence for it multiple times before it is learned by a client.

PUTTING IT ALL TOGETHER

Although the specific therapeutic strategies discussed above may seem straightforward, their actual application can feel confusing and chaotic to family therapists, particularly when therapists reach out to families who do not come into a clinic weekly for family therapy sessions. The players change; the issues change; families cut off contact; and clients reappear in a different family configuration after a crisis.

The following case illustrates the episodic and changing nature of proactive intervention. It also shows how useful it is to have consistent goals throughout. Although the case is a composite of several cases to protect confidentiality, every aspect reflects actual client issues, actual therapist responses, and actual client outcomes.

Case Example

Richard Heath (age 14), his sister, Jean Heath (age 12), and their mother, Mrs. Sonya Procino (age 31), were referred by the children's guidance counselor to a therapist for community-based family therapy. Richard was repeating seventh grade after having received F's in all his five major subjects. The guidance counselor was concerned that even with a different set of teachers, he had again gotten F's in all major subjects during the first two grading periods of the current school year. The guidance counselor's concerns about Jean were that she cried frequently and that some of her comments expressed suicidal ideation (i.e., she wished she were dead).

The school's Child Study Team had recommended counseling for Richard previously because of his poor grades and frequent fighting at school, but Mrs. Procino had not pursued this option. The guidance counselor got the mother's permission to refer them this time, for several reasons: (1) Mrs. Procino trusted her because she had supported her in her efforts to get off welfare and into a job; (2) the counseling could be done at school and in their home; and (3) there would be no cost to the mother, who had no health insurance, because a grant paid for the services.

Family History

Mrs. Procino grew up in the same small, working class, predominantly European American town where she currently lived in a rented house with Mr. Procino (who was disabled), Richard, Jean, and their 6-year-old half-brother, Jim. Mrs. Procino escaped from the responsibilities of caring for her schizophrenic, Italian-speaking mother, her abusive, alcoholic father, and her four younger siblings when she became pregnant with Richard at 16 and was taken to another state by Mr. Heath. When Richard and Jean were 3 and 1½ years old, respectively, Mrs. Procino left their father because of his physical abuse. Although she returned to the town of her birth, Mrs. Procino fended for herself until she met Mr. Procino, who took care of the children while she worked. She still did not communicate with her father or mother, as she feared that she would be drawn back into taking care of them. One by one, each of her siblings had left their parents' home and pointedly stayed out of contact, apparently for the same reason.

Assessment

Mrs. Procino and Jim came in after school one Monday afternoon and met with the therapist and Richard and Jean, after the therapist had first met separately with the two older siblings. Because Mrs. Procino's job (laundering sheets and towels) was on the "graveyard shift," meetings could only be scheduled on Mondays, because her sleeping hours were more regular on weekends.

Mrs. Procino, an extremely heavy woman, was loud, very critical, and demanding with her children. She did all of the talking unless she or the therapist asked her children a question. At one point during the initial interview, she swatted Jim hard on his behind and yelled, "Sit down!" when he got out of his seat and began wandering around the classroom. Although the therapist had report cards and teachers' comments stating that Richard did no homework, the therapist decided that his initial session would focus on Mrs. Procino, so that she would see that attending sessions had immediate "payoffs" for her. Therefore, the conversation centered on how the children "did not pay any attention" to their mother, how they "stayed out late after curfew," and how they "did not do their chores."

The first goal, even before learning about the family history, was geared to Mrs. Procino's greatest problem—getting the children to do their chores. The therapist led them through the problem-solving steps about how chores could get done. A list was made of which child was responsible for what chores, and it was agreed (to the children's relief) that they were responsible for doing chores only on Saturdays, instead of every day, as their mother had previously demanded.

The therapist continued to see Richard and Jean separately each week in school to learn more about them. They each wanted more freedom. Richard's "dream" was to be a professional football player; Jean's was to be a nurse. It also became clear that there were frequent name-calling and hitting episodes among the siblings, particularly when they ordered each other to do things. For instance, Richard would yell, "Jean, get your fat butt in here and give Jim his dinner." Jean was especially sensitive to such insults because she, like her mother, had a weight problem. Jean would hit Richard or Jim, and Richard would beat up Jean until she said, "I give up."

In addition to not handing in any homework, Richard's teachers reported that he did not do any classwork. Richard could not explain his behavior to the therapist, and so (with his and the teacher's permission), the therapist sat through one of Richard's math classes. He saw him staring out of the window, sharpening his pencil, and talking to the students next to him and in front of him, but doing no deskwork.

During this time, the therapist also worked with the whole family at home. When Mr. and Mrs. Procino expressed concern about Richard's curfew violations, the therapist asked Mr. Procino, who was at home at curfew time, to keep a weekly record of when Richard came home in preparation for a future problem-solving session.

During another session, 1 month after the first, Mrs. Procino, Richard, Jean, Jim, and the therapist agreed upon the following goals for Richard and Jean:

1. That they receive at least D's—an improvement from F's—in all of their courses.
2. That they receive less detention and fewer school suspensions.

3. That they do chores at home without being reminded more than
   once.
4. That they continue to be home by their curfews.
5. That they hit each other less often.
6. That they talk about their lives to their parents.

Case Formulation

It appeared that Richard had learned to wait to be directed by his
mother (or another adult) to do things, rather than risk being told he
was doing things wrong. He did not initiate difficult activity, such as
schoolwork. Instead, by staying away from the house for as long as he
could, he had learned to pursue what he found to be pleasurable activities: stealing jewelry and using alcohol and drugs.

Jean, on the other hand, did not have friends or places to go. She
stayed home and cleaned and cooked, trying vainly to get praise from
her parents and younger brother. She had developed a habit of telling
herself all her faults before her mother could tell her what was wrong
with her. She was also the victim of family recreational "wrestling"
matches, which other family members rationalized as being helpful
because they "made her stronger."

Both older children needed more prosocial mastery experiences,
especially in their deficient areas—academics for Richard and social
interaction for Jean. The mother was powerful, hard-working, and committed. She managed to provide her children with an income and a clean
house; however, she could not help them with schoolwork because she
had not completed school herself, and could not check that they kept
their curfews because she was at work. From her own childhood experiences, she had learned beliefs and practices about parenting that put her
children at risk. For example, she felt she needed to point out everything
they did wrong, rather than what they did right; she gave orders and
never helped her children to think for themselves; she believed that her
daughter was "out to get me" and needed to be toughened up, without
realizing that Jean looked to her mother for guidance and approval; she
believed her kids misbehaved only because of their treatment at the
hands of their biological father; and she was convinced that the principal
wanted her kids out of his school.

Intervention: Positive Feedback from the Environment

Because Mrs. Procino was very concerned about being a good mother,
she responded positively to repeated recognition from the therapist
about how much she did for her children. After the therapist communi-

cated respect for Mrs. Procino, she was more willing to consider the therapist's ideas about child rearing. Whenever possible, the therapist would intervene with alternative suggestions for Mrs. Procino:

> "Let your children know when you see them doing something good, like completing their homework or making curfew."
>
> "The kids are learning how to be people by watching you and Mr. Procino right now. Especially, your daughter needs you to guide her on how to be a woman. I think she's too developed to be wrestling with the family any more, don't you?"
>
> "To help the kids learn to think for themselves instead of being followers, ask them, 'What are you going to do to solve this problem?,' instead of telling them what to do."
>
> "I understand you need to discipline Jim, but I'm afraid he's learning from you to hit his friends when he wants them to do something."

New Role Models

The therapist continued to meet with Richard and Jean individually each week, focusing on problem solving, day-to-day schoolwork, recreational activities, and social relations. Before these meetings, he would see one of their teachers to learn about their assignments. He was instrumental in helping Richard to surmount several obstacles to play on a recreational basketball team that was coached by one of his teachers. He often discussed Richard's sports achievements with the teacher and supported the teacher for the extra efforts that he made for Richard, such as driving him home.

After learning that the school nurse had included Jean in a weight-monitoring program, the therapist spoke to the nurse about Jean's circumstances. As a result, the nurse chose Jean to be one of her student assistants. These three periods each week provided Jean with much-needed attention and acknowledgment.

Monitoring

Even though Richard was complying with his curfew more often and getting recognition for this from Mr. Procino, he was caught with some stolen jewelry and given a court date. Mr. and Mrs. Procino were shocked and began learning more about the adolescents Richard spent time with. With the therapist's guidance, they began to address with Richard whether it was in his interest to spend time with some of his "friends." Both parents were careful to give Richard time to respond and reach his own conclusions, rather than imposing their own judgments on him.

Changing Beliefs

Besides suggesting alternative beliefs to Mrs. Procino about child rearing, the therapist also made suggestions to the children as to how they might change their negative beliefs. Although her mother's castigations had diminished, Jean still frequently felt hurt and rejected. The therapist helped Jean to see that her mother's criticisms might be more a function of her mother's life stress and tiredness than of Jean's "badness." The counselor also constantly asked each child, when he or she was angry about something, "Can you think of something to do about it that won't hurt *you?*"

The therapist spent almost a whole school year searching for a motivation that would result in Richard's doing more schoolwork. Neither getting out of middle school before he was 16 nor being able to play football in high school seemed to motivate him. One day, however, he announced in a weekly individual session that he had completed the achievement tests that would determine whether he could do ninth grade work. When asked by the therapist, "How did you get yourself to do that?," he replied, "I realized that if I just go ahead and do this, then I'll get it over with." The therapist was able to say quite genuinely, "Now, that's an idea!" because Richard had generated it on his own. Richard went on to finish eighth grade with enough passing grades to go to high school.

Increasing Adult Involvement in the Adolescents' Lives

The first areas in which the therapist helped involve the parents were peers, curfews, and schoolwork. After the parents showed more awareness of what their children were doing in these areas, the therapist worked with the parents to promote activities for Richard and Jean that would be actively positive. The school informed the therapist of a small, federally funded job program in the town. Richard was old enough and was automatically eligible because of his special education status. Thus he had an interested set of adults who had no preconceived notions about him guide him through his first (and successful) employment experience.

During a follow-up, booster-session phone call, the mother acknowledged to the therapist that her kids were doing more things she wanted them to without her having to tell them to. She attributed the improvement to her children's learning "how to behave from you and

Mr. Procino and their peers." The therapist quickly said, "It's also because you're now acknowledging them when you see them doing what you want, and because you're asking, 'What are you going to do about that?' instead of trying to solve their problems for them."

In Richard's last session, the therapist talked more frankly about the boy's alcohol and drug use than he had done before. He said, "Even though you say your use is causing you no trouble now, one day you may want to stop. Carry my telephone number with you and call me if you ever want to talk."

Long-Term Outcome

Despite the short-term gains, Richard dropped out of school soon after he was 16. He had not been able to play football in high school because his mother did not give him permission and because his grades were not good enough. His sister, however, became an assistant to the high school nurse and stayed in school.

One and a half years after their last session, Richard left the following message on the therapist's answering machine: "You were right. I need drug rehab." Following this call, the therapist helped Richard get into an outpatient program. He learned that he had left home because of fighting with his mother and was living with an aunt to whom Mrs. Procino did not speak. The therapist also learned that the impetus for Richard's phone call was probably that he had just been arrested for dealing cocaine.

The therapist gradually engaged the aunt and then a second aunt in Richard's counseling. The aunts began talking to each other for the first time, and to Richard, about the abuse they each had experienced from their father and about their helplessness and guilt about their schizophrenic mother.

After much respectful persistence by the therapist, Mrs. Procino and all of her siblings met several times with Richard; they also began to make plans for their now terminally ill father and still psychotic mother. After four difficult, intense sessions with the community-based therapist, they all began going to Richard's aftercare program for further family meetings. Richard's active participation in therapy and in evening school persuaded the judge to put him on probation instead of in prison.

PART III

SCHOOL AND COMMUNITY WORK

CHAPTER 7

Working with Schools and Preschools

Schools and preschools are integral elements of outreach work with children and families. We recommend working closely with the schools for various reasons: First, therapists can work more confidently when they have objective evidence regarding children's outcomes, such as improved grades. Second, teachers can become a valuable part of the change process. Improvement occurs faster, because positive changes in teachers' evaluations of students can be acknowledged while negative changes can lead to immediate intervention.

School behavior is often indicative of other problems in children's and adolescents' lives (Loeber, 1990). Furthermore, Dryfoos (1990) concludes that school performance is the single greatest predictor of children's futures. In one home- and school-based treatment outcome study (Krinsley, 1991), not one of the seventh- or eighth-graders who received individual and family counseling for 4 months initiated or increased drug use either during the intervention or during the succeeding school year. This result was achieved even though schoolwork, not drug use, was the focus of the intervention. School is the equivalent of a workplace for children and adolescents. If they learn how to handle its challenges, they will be able to handle employment later on. Likewise, knowing that they can do well in school buffers adolescents from the effects of stress outside of school (Wills, Blechman, & McNamara, 1996).

This chapter begins with a discussion of the important challenges of confidentiality issues a therapist may encounter when working with schools, preschools, and other agencies. It also includes brief sections on working with preschools and elementary schools, but it focuses primarily on middle and high schools. Because middle and high schools usually have many more students, heightened security needs, and privacy concerns, it is often more difficult for a parent or family worker to enter, identify key personnel, and develop a reliable method for following a student's progress. Our discussion of secondary schools also includes a section on prevention work with at-risk adolescents in these schools. Prevention is an integral element of outreach, and therapists have an opportunity to work most effectively when they bring their programs to the students and their families through the schools. The chapter concludes with a summary of lessons we have learned from our work; these guidelines should facilitate the work of all therapists who have even very limited contact with schools.

CONFIDENTIALITY WITH SCHOOLS, PRESCHOOLS, AND OTHER AGENCIES

The rules of confidentiality that are applicable to clinical work clearly apply here as well. *Therapists should get written permission from the parents to contact any schools (within which the therapists are not working) and other agencies that may be involved with the family* (Bry & Greene, 1988–1989). A distinction needs to be made in this context between getting and giving information. Although therapists should obtain from referral sources and other agencies as much information as they have available, therapists should be careful to give only information that benefits the client. They should also be vigilant about the tone of their reports about clients. Therapists or family workers are human and often become frustrated with particular clients or families; this frustration may inadvertently influence the way in which they discuss or write about their clients.

Schools and preschools are understandably eager to get feedback from family workers regarding the progress of children or adolescents and their families. We have found that even a simple statement by a family worker that a family and a child (or adolescent) are participating in treatment can influence positively the way in which the family and the child (or adolescent) are viewed by the school (Bry & Greene, 1988–1989). This may communicate to the teachers and school officials that the family and the child (adolescent) are "trying," and thus it may engender more support for them. Again, however, unless the therapist works in the schools, no information can be given to schools without the express permission of the child and family.

PRESCHOOLS AND DAY CARE PROGRAMS

As shown in Chapter 5, very young children are frequently referred for treatment. If a child is already in a day care or preschool program, the therapist should incorporate the school into the intervention. A combined "reaching-out" intervention will aim to meet with the staff at the day care center or preschool, and with the family at either the school or the family home, as in the case of Billy in Chapter 5 (Billy's case is discussed further below). School-linked, home-based services play an important role in promoting children's well-being (Black & Krishnakumar, 1998).

As stated in Chapter 5, sometimes the role of the family therapist involves helping a parent who is overwhelmed with many young children at home to find a good day care or preschool program. This need is especially severe in the case of parents who, due to recent federal legislation, are required to participate in the workforce through "Welfare to Work" or "Work First" programs. Although parents are often given vouchers for day care, there are few slots and long waiting lists for the best programs. A family worker or agency familiar with preschool programs can often facilitate this process.

A child may also be referred by the day care center or preschool. Aggressiveness toward other children and adults, sexually inappropriate behavior, or concerns about serious developmental delays can often lead to referrals, even at this young age. Rickel and Becker (1997) make a strong case that effective intervention at this age can change the trajectory of the rest of a child's life for the better.

When family therapists have received a referral from a day care center for a child who is acting out, fighting with other children, sexually inappropriate, or extremely depressed or withdrawn, it is often helpful for the family therapist to meet with the center director and the teacher(s). The next step might involve meeting with the family at the preschool or day care program. In some cases, it is also helpful for the family worker to observe the child in his or her classroom and consult with the teacher on behavior management strategies.

Case Example

Billy was referred by his day care program because he had recently seemed very angry, had been hitting other children, and often threw temper tantrums when asked to perform routine activities. His mother was having a great deal of difficulty managing his behavior since her separation from his father 2 months previously (see Chapter 5 for a complete description of this family).

In addition to the family treatment, the therapist met (with the mother's permission) with Billy's preschool teacher and her assistant. Both were very fond of Billy, but were concerned about his aggressiveness. Other children were refusing to play with him, and there had been complaints from other parents because of Billy's behavior.

After getting permission to observe Billy in his preschool class, the therapist sat in the back of the room for approximately 40 minutes. In that time, Billy snatched one child's snack, hit another boy and took his truck, and angrily said "No!" and ran away when the classroom aide tried to stop him.

The therapist worked with the teachers to develop a behavior management program that would help Billy and his classmates. She helped the teachers to establish a "time-out room" in a small anteroom outside the classroom. It was agreed that if hitting behavior occurred, the teachers would say firmly (not angrily) to Billy or any other child, "No, hitting is not allowed. You will have to go to time out. You can come back when you can behave." A kitchen timer would then be set for 5 minutes, and the child would be placed in the anteroom without toys and other playthings, after which he or she would be returned to the classroom.

The therapist worked with the teachers to emphasize the power of positive reinforcement for Billy. They were encouraged to "catch him being good" and to praise him. Also, a "sticker system" was instituted for the whole group. A chart was made for the class, and after each activity, anyone who had done well received a check. At the end of the day, each child with four or more checks was allowed to choose a sticker to paste in a notebook. Billy and all of the other children loved this exercise and worked hard to earn this reward.

In Billy's case, these were coordinated with a similar system at home. His mother agreed that as soon as he got five stickers in his notebook, they would spend a special "mommy–son" afternoon at the park. It took Billy about 3 weeks to earn this, but he worked hard, and his behavior in class began to improve. "Time out" had to be used twice in the first week and once in the second week, but in the third week he had not hit another child.

Discussion

This case illustrates the ways in which therapists can work closely with day care or preschool programs to target difficult or disruptive behaviors and develop a behavior management program. A point system or "sticker system" is very useful with this age group. Immediate reinforcement through a check on the class chart after a successful activity is important, because preschool children need such reinforcement. Colorful stickers and colored stars can be obtained inexpensively in bulk. Teachers and parents should be encouraged to make a "big deal" out of these rewards and to praise each successful activity. It is very helpful to coordinate this with a similar practice at home (Dishion & Patterson, 1996). Parents and teachers working together with the therapist can be a powerful motivational system.

ELEMENTARY SCHOOLS

A wide range of behavioral and learning difficulties may be identified for the first time when children begin school. Problems may include conduct disorder, oppositional defiant disorder, anxiety, depression, grief reactions, learning difficulties, and school failure. It is our belief that even if a referral is for a family or individual problem seemingly unrelated to school, permission should be obtained from a parent to contact the school for information. Because children and adolescents spend so many hours in schools, assessing their school behavior is an extremely important part of assessing their overall functioning (Henggeler et al., 1998).

An area of concern to parents and teachers in recent years has been the growing number of elementary school children referred for learning disabilities and attention-deficit/hyperactivity disorder (ADHD). The initial presenting problem is often that the children appear to be failing or underachieving in school. These children present a puzzle to their parents and teachers: Although they seem bright and have strengths in certain academic areas, they are not able to absorb one or more vital components of instruction (such as math, reading, or writing), or they have problems with visual, auditory, or language processing or comprehension (Barkley, 1998). Children who have ADHD may also have trouble attending, concentrating, sitting still in class, remembering their assignments, retaining ideas and concepts from one day to the next, and organizing their work and bookbags (Barkley, 1995). These children are often distractible and can miss a class lecture or assignment because they are paying attention to something outside their classroom.

The following case illustrates how a child diagnosed with ADHD and his family were guided by a family therapist through the process of getting help. It also shows how workers need to balance mental health considerations with other significant issues that confront minority families (Boyd-Franklin, 1989).

Case Example

Kwame was a 10-year-old African American boy who was referred for treatment by his fifth-grade teacher. His father, Walter Hanes (age 37), was a truck driver; his mother, Dorothy Hanes (age 35), was a waitress. His younger brother, Nyere, a 7-year-old second-grader, was regarded by everyone in the family as the "good child." He got all A's and behaved well in school and at home. Kwame was "the problem." His teacher reported that he was bright but "did not try hard enough." She would often catch him daydreaming in school, with no idea of what the class was learning. He also "could not sit still" and was constantly twirling a pencil, opening and closing his desk, teasing and distracting other children, or getting out of his seat and walking around the classroom. In short, he seemed to be in "perpetual motion."

Kwame's parents reported that he was "lazy" and often lied about not having any homework. They described him as a "pistol" and "hell on wheels" at home. His mother reported that the two boys were constantly fighting; Kwame picked on and teased his brother. He also had a very short attention span. The longest period of concentration he had demonstrated was the 4- to 6-minute span in which he could play the video games he loved.

The school had recommended psychological testing and an evaluation by the Child Study Team (CST). Mr. and Mrs. Hanes, like many African American parents, were very skeptical about the school's motives and approached each suggestion with a large dose of the "healthy cultural suspicion" discussed in Chapter 2 (Boyd-Franklin, 1989; Grier & Cobbs, 1968). Mrs. Hanes expressed the concern that the school system was trying to "label my child." Mr. Hanes was very angry because he felt that Black boys are disproportionately referred for CST evaluations and placement in special education programs. This is an accurate and common concern among Black parents, and hence they are often skeptical when schools make such recommendations (Kunjufu, 1985). The therapist agreed with the parents that this often happens to Black male children and praised them for their vigilance on Kwame's behalf.

The therapist, an African American social worker at a community mental health center, met first with the entire family in her office. Nyere sat very close to his parents, while Kwame was in constant motion during the session. He fidgeted, teased his brother, talked out of turn, and sampled most of the toys in the therapist's toy corner. Initially Mr. Hanes yelled at him to sit down, but eventually he seemed to give up and ignored him.

The parents' frustration with Kwame and with the school was apparent immediately. Mr. Hanes was insistent in his skepticism about therapy, testing, and other psychological interventions. The therapist worked hard to join with both parents as well as with Kwame and Nyere in the first session. She explored the parents' concerns about the psychological testing, as well as about the meeting with a psychiatrist and neurologist that the Child Study Team had requested. Mr. Hanes refused to have his child evaluated by the school. With the parents' permission on a signed consent form, the therapist agreed to call the school. But before she had the opportunity to do so, Mrs. Hanes called to say that Kwame had been suspended for fighting. What had started out with name calling resulted in another boy's hitting Kwame and Kwame's hitting back. Both boys were suspended pending a meeting with their parents. With the parents' permission, the therapist called the school and asked to attend that meeting.

Prior to the meeting, the therapist obtained permission to make a school visit and met with Kwame's teacher, his guidance counselor, and the school's principal. The principal was very concerned for Kwame and seemed to want to help him, but she insisted that Kwame would not be allowed to return to school unless the parents agreed to the testing and the rest of the Child Study Team's evaluation. All of the school personnel the therapist spoke with reported that they "could not deal" with Mr. Hanes because of his eruptions of anger during their meetings with him.

The therapist decided to meet with Mr. and Mrs. Hanes to discuss this issue prior to the school meeting. When she discussed the school's position, Mr. Hanes initially became angry. The therapist empathized with his concern for his son and asked him whether he could see any way around this dilemma. Both parents were silent. The therapist then asked the parents whether they would consider having an independent psychological testing done at the community mental health center. Initially Mr. Hanes was opposed to this also, but finally he and his wife agreed to this as a compromise.

The therapist then called the principal and the head of the Child Study Team to explore this possibility. Although both were resistant at first to this break with protocol, they agreed because of their concerns for Kwame. The meeting the following week at the school was, by all reports, the most productive session Mr. and Mrs. Hanes had ever had with school officials. Although both sides were initially guarded, the therapist was able to help them discuss the issues together. They reached a compromise where it was agreed that Kwame would be seen for psychological testing and educational testing at the clinic. The therapist, as a social worker, would be allowed to contribute the psychosocial portion of the evaluation. The head of the Child Study Team emphasized throughout the unusualness of this procedure, and maintained that she and the other members of the team retained the right to review all materials and develop the final recommendations and Individualized Educational Plan (IEP) for Kwame.

The therapist continued to work with Mr. and Mrs. Hanes, Kwame, and Nyere in family therapy sessions. She had gained their trust and had increasing credibility with them. She helped them develop strategies for managing the behavior of both boys at home, such as keeping a "star chart" on which good behavior was rewarded. The therapist also worked with the teacher on some behavior management techniques for the classroom.

The evaluation process at the community mental health center identified learning disabilities in the areas of language processing, math, and reading. The psychologist and learning specialist also agreed that Kwame had ADHD and recommended that he be placed on the medication Ritalin. Mr. and Mrs. Hanes were both furious when they received this feedback. Mrs. Hanes explained that their worst fears had been realized: Kwame had been "labeled" and was being "put on drugs." The therapist sympathized with the parents' concerns and asked them how much they knew about learning disabilities and ADHD. They reported that they had seen articles in popular magazines talking about "overmedication" of children on Ritalin. They discussed their concerns openly. With the therapist's help, they made a list of all of their questions. These were addressed subsequently in several weeks of family therapy and education (see Barkley, 1998).

After 3 months, the school asked Kwame's parents to attend a parent conference with the Child Study Team, to which the therapist was also invited. The head of the team summarized the results of the evaluation and recommended that Kwame be placed in a regular class with a resource room. She also strongly recommended that the family place Kwame on a trial of Ritalin. Mr. Hanes became very angry and stormed out of the meeting. The next day Kwame got involved in a fight in the cafeteria with several other children and was again suspended. It was clear that Kwame's behavior had escalated. The principal and the head of the Child Study Team were adamant that he could not return to school unless the team's recommendations were implemented.

When the therapist met with the parents, Mr. Hanes was slumped in his chair, and both he and Mrs. Hanes looked defeated. Desperately searching for a compromise, the therapist asked the parents whether they would consider a 3-month trial of the team's plan, including the Ritalin. The therapist agreed to work closely with the parents and the school on behavior management strategies during that time. She told the parents not to answer right away, but to think about it and give her an answer in their next session. Two days before the scheduled session, Ms. Hanes called to say that she and her husband had decided to try it.

The next week, Kwame was placed on Ritalin. The therapist had prepared the parents and Kwame for the possibility that the medication might have to be adjusted many times until the right dosage was found and he was free of side effects. The therapist also made arrangements for the parents to meet the resource room teacher at the school prior to Kwame's reentry. She helped to develop an alliance between the parents and the new teacher, and arranged to "check in" with the teacher by phone once per week. Another parent–teacher meeting was scheduled for the end of the marking period (2 months later).

After an initial period in which Kwame's dosage of Ritalin was first too low and then too high, the correct dosage was found. Because the family had been prepared for this possibility by the therapist, they were able to accept the adjustment process. By the end of the first month, Kwame's homeroom teacher, his resource room teacher, and his guidance counselor reported a great deal of improvement. The counselor said that the change was "very dramatic." She stated that she had observed Kwame in the classroom and he was able to sit still and attend to the lesson. He seemed to take great pride in being able to raise his hand when appropriate and answer questions correctly.

In family sessions, his parents and Nyere expressed similar reactions. The therapist was careful to give Kwame's parents the credit in the session for being willing to "take the chances necessary to help your son." She praised them for all of the "agonizing" they had done "out of love and concern for your son" and for advocating on his behalf. Both parents beamed proudly and were in turn able to praise Kwame directly for his success in school. Mrs. Hanes reported that she had always known her son was bright, and that now she could see his abilities coming through.

At the end of the marking period, the scheduled conference was held with the parents, the therapist, Kwame, the classroom teacher, the resource room teacher, the guidance counselor, the head of the Child Study Team, and the principal. Everyone praised Kwame for excellent work. The mood was much lighter. It was wonderful to see the transformation in all family members and school personnel at this meeting.

At the end of the school year, Kwame passed all of his subjects and received the "most improved student" award at the final assembly.

Discussion

This case clearly illustrates the value of school-based sessions and the role of the therapist in serving as a mediator and facilitator between the family and the school. It was important that the therapist recognize the parents' cultural and racial concerns for their son. Because of her successful joining with the members of this family, her understanding of their cultural concerns and her willingness to reach out to the school, the therapist was able to help all parties find a viable solution for Kwame.

MIDDLE AND HIGH SCHOOLS

Prevention

Bry and her associates have shown that preventive intervention programs for youth whom schools identify as "high-risk" can make a difference in reducing future drug and alcohol abuse, academic failure, and juvenile delinquency (Alexander, 1997; Bry, 1982; Bry, Conboy, & Bisgay, 1986; Bry & George, 1980; Bry & Krinsley, 1992; Krinsley, 1991). One of Bry's prevention programs, the Early Secondary Intervention Program (ESIP), has been placed by the U.S. Department of Education (under the name of "Bry's Behavioral Monitoring and Reinforcement Program") on its list of empirically supported interventions. The Early Secondary Intervention Program entails weekly counseling for selected high-risk youth in the schools, and monthly outreach phone calls or visits to their homes to keep parents informed about their children's progress at school. (See Stanley, Goldstein, & Bry, 1976.) Bry's second program, Targeted Family Intervention (TFI), begins with weekly school-based individual counseling; it then adds coordinated weekly home-based family therapy sessions in order to increase preventive effects. (See Bry et al., 1991.)

Some examples of "warning signs" that schools can use to identify high-risk youth as they move into middle school are the following: an increase in school absences and suspensions; increased school failure due to poor skills and/or motivation to complete work; greater experience of reprimands in school; and lack of participation in conventional extracurricular activities (Bry, 1996). At the same time, these youth often simultaneously experience increasing success and appreciation in the company of older school dropouts, who in high drug-trafficking neighborhoods may be using and/or dealing drugs (Gottfredson & Hirschi, 1994). For African American and other minority youth, particularly in low-income communities, there is also an increased risk of violence, gang involvement, teenage pregnancy, and the collective effects of racism and discrimination (National Research Council, 1993; Taylor & Wang, 1997).

Parker (1995) has shown that parents of high-risk adolescents, despite their best efforts, often feel powerless to guide their children away from conduct problems and school failure. These parents' good intentions can be overwhelmed by the pervasive internal and external stressors of their existence, such as poverty, social and cultural isolation, depression, physical illness, poor communication and persuasion skills, a high-crime environment engendering fear, and lack of knowledge of their children's high-risk activities (Parece, 1997). Research has shown, however, that early identification and intervention can help parents reduce risk factors that interfere with the lives of high-risk adolescents (Bry & Alexander, 1997).

Early intervention with high-risk adolescents and their families necessarily involves (1) proactively gaining access to the youth and their families through reaching out to them, instead of waiting for them to come regularly to a clinic for help; and (2) assertively applying resources and energy to change the relationship between them and some of the multiple systems that affect their lives. In order for a prevention program to be effective, family therapists need to know the following: with whom to intervene; where to contact adolescents who need intervention; what goals to target; specific intervention strategies; and a means for assessing whether or not goals are attained. We have found that working with the schools is useful because schools can identify which adolescents need help; schools are where adolescents are located; school officials can help to persuade parents to agree to the interventions; school records contain the information that we need; and schools can provide feedback, a source for evaluating our effectiveness.

We realize that most family therapists do not have to identify whom to treat, since clients come to them already selected. Once selection takes place, however, many of the challenges of prevention work, such as how to approach and collaborate with school staff, are shared by family therapists working with an adolescent population.

Selecting High-Risk Adolescents

Empirical evidence shows that adolescents with early warning signs such as truancy, poor grades, conduct problems, and family conflict have an increased probability of developing severe problems later on, such as substance abuse, delinquency, and/or school dropout (Bry, 1996; Bry, McKeon, & Pandina, 1982; Loeber, 1990). It is preferable to intervene with younger adolescents who already show these risk factors but who do not yet have severe problems. We have found that the seventh and eighth grades are good points at which to identify youngsters in danger of repeating a grade because of academic failure, poor attendance, or a level of discipline referrals that brings detention and suspension. The goal is to reduce these risk factors, on the assumption that the probability of severe problems will likewise be reduced (Bry & Greene, 1990).

Approaching the Schools

Schools are systems that are, by law, self-contained and self-sufficient. They have their own psychologists and social workers, and they are responsible for, and must portray themselves as adequately meeting, all of the educational needs of their students. This presents a challenge for outsiders.

Some schools may block family workers' efforts in preventive intervention. There are, however, at least three conditions that make entry possible:

1. Family workers should be introduced to a school administrator—a principal or superintendent—by someone the administrator trusts. The process of maintaining relationships with the schools is continuous, for school personnel continually change.

2. The school administrator must be willing to admit that some children's needs are not being met by currently available resources.

3. Assuming entry is permitted, school personnel must be convinced that their work is facilitated rather than complicated by the family workers' presence. They should not have to fill out even one extra sheet of paper or take even one more phone call from an irate parent because of the prevention program. Instead, family therapists should work to ensure that school staff members feel relieved that the therapists have come, because the therapists can address some of the children's needs that the school personnel have been unable to address themselves.

Approaching Adolescents and Their Families

Once a school agrees to a prevention program, the family therapists talk with the school's personnel—the principal(s), guidance counselor(s), Child Study Team, nurse, and teachers—about the risk factors. To preserve confidentiality, the school personnel look at the records to identify high-risk students. Then they contact the selected adolescents and parents and ask their permission to enroll them in the prevention program. The principal writes the initial letter, and a guidance counselor follows up with a phone call. In addition to preserving the confidentiality of the school records until parents give permission for a therapist to work with the adolescent, this method of selection and recruitment increases the acceptance rate, since parents know the school personnel and do not yet know the family therapist.

The way in which school personnel describe the project also affects the acceptance rate. They should phrase their approach to adolescents and parents in a positive manner: They should state that they see these youth as "students who can do better in school." This is usually a new, surprising message for the parents of high-risk adolescents to get from the school. (Most of these parents are used to getting critical messages.) A positive emphasis encourages an affirmative response.

The acceptance rate for the Targeted Family Intervention is 88%. That is, 88% of the identified high-risk adolescents' families agree, and of those, 100% stay in the program (Krinsley, 1991)! This figure usually astonishes people, for many of these families have been referred to mental health services in the past, and they did not go. Henggeler, Pickrel, Brondino, and Crouch (1996) have also succeeded in eliminating dropout in their home-based multisystemic therapy, which employs many methods similar to ours. We characterize our own approach to recruiting adolescents and families as "respectfully persistent and patient." We do not expect enthusiasm or initiative on their part. After all, the notion that an intervention could be useful is our idea—not theirs.

Once a parent agrees that a child can participate in the intervention, a family therapist goes to the school and is introduced to the adolescent by the guidance counselor. The therapist engages the adolescent in a few minutes of pleasant conversation. Next, the therapist counsels the student individually in school for a few weeks in order to establish trust. This technique decreases the chance that the adolescent will discourage the parent from meeting with the family therapist.

Then the family therapist calls the parents and asks to meet with them to learn the parents' views about what could help their adolescent do better in school and stay out of trouble. Parents often have a lot of ideas, and, again, are pleasantly surprised to be asked. The therapist offers to meet with the parents in their home, at the school, or at the office. Quite frequently, scheduled meetings are changed, canceled, or forgotten by the parents. If so, the family therapist respectfully and persistently schedules another. Meanwhile, the therapist can go on meeting with the adolescent at school.

Proactive Intervention with Adolescents

Once permission is granted to intervene with adolescents, we have found that therapists' first challenge is to demonstrate that the intervention will not bring any negative consequences to the adolescents. Adolescents can be amazingly cooperative if they believe that no harm will be done. They also can easily sabotage others' support of family therapists by disparaging the therapists to their parents or teachers. In order to prevent the risk that adolescents will ask authority figures to withdraw permission for the intervention (which many parents will do if their adolescents request it), the therapist ideally should demonstrate to adolescents that it will bring immediate benefits.

Practitioners in proactive early intervention programs need attitudes, policies, and approaches that are very different from the "passive-receptive" stance of office-bound therapists who have clients with "felt needs." Early intervention is the practitioners' idea, not the adolescents' or the families', as was pointed out above. Consequently, practitioners carry 99% of the responsibility for initiating sessions, and ensuring that they happen, for the duration of the intervention. It is often a therapist alone who believes that an adolescent can do better in school and get into less trouble, and it is often a therapist alone who believes that counseling can bring about that improvement.

We think of our intervention program as a "no-dropout" program. Common reasons given for dropping an adolescent from a "passive-receptive" intervention, such as that the adolescent "is not motivated," "is not taking advantage of the program," or "does not want to meet with the practitioner," do not influence the continuation or cessation of our intervention. As long as a practitioner knows that the intervention will benefit an adolescent, he or she takes responsibility for continuing to reach out. As we have noted above, we characterize our own stance as being "respectfully persistent." It also could be characterized as "caring."

Working with the Schools

A family therapist who has obtained a signed release-of-information form from a parent can have access to up-to-date, accurate information about an adolescent from the school. We interview a different one of the adolescent's teachers once a week and copy the attendance and discipline information. Ideally, the family therapists interview the teachers. Some programs, however, have found it useful to hire a part-time para-professional to spend 1 day a week in the schools, interviewing the teachers and filling out Weekly Report Cards on each student, which the therapists can discuss during therapy sessions. (See Weekly Report Card in Figure 7.1.) The personal interview is far superior to having teachers fill out the forms. Forms would mean extra paperwork for the teachers, and their tendency is to provide fairly negative and vague information while filling out forms, instead of the positive, specific information that therapists need.

Official quarterly report cards are also a valuable source of infor-

WEEKLY REPORT CARD

Student: _____ Therapist: _____ Date: _____

Did this student do these things *during the past week?*

TEACHER	GET TO CLASS ON TIME?	BRING MATERIALS FOR CLASS?	DO CLASSWORK?	RECENT GRADES	SHOW SATISFACTORY BEHAVIOR?	DO HOMEWORK?	WAS HOMEWORK ASSIGNED?	DATE
	YES NO	YES NO	YES NO		YES NO	YES NO	YES NO	
	YES NO	YES NO	YES NO		YES NO	YES NO	YES NO	
	YES NO	YES NO	YES NO		YES NO	YES NO	YES NO	
	YES NO	YES NO	YES NO		YES NO	YES NO	YES NO	
	YES NO	YES NO	YES NO		YES NO	YES NO	YES NO	
	YES NO	YES NO	YES NO		YES NO	YES NO	YES NO	
	YES NO	YES NO	YES NO		YES NO	YES NO	YES NO	

Assignments that student should be working on: _____

Other comments: _____

Dates of absences: _____

Dates and reasons for discipline referrals: _____

FIGURE 7.1. Weekly Report Card.

mation. To interpret outcomes, however, therapists must realize that success in preventive interventions with high-risk adolescents is often demonstrated when grades remain at the same level or even when they decrease slightly. This is because without the intervention, high-risk adolescents' grades and attendance tend to decline markedly every year (Bry & George, 1980). Because of this, to assess success, a family therapist working with the school needs to compare a student's official report card with last year's or with that of a similar high-risk student who was not in the preventive intervention.

Prevention practitioners must remember that regardless of the nobility of their motives, parents and teachers will work with them only if they experience their efforts as making their own jobs easier rather than harder. Teachers, in particular, have a myriad of experiences with new programs that demand disproportionately extra work on their part and provide little payoff for them or their students. It becomes a survival skill for them to avoid such unplanned work. Thus, by the time family therapists come along, teachers may be skeptical, wary, and practiced at avoiding what they perceive to be well-meaning but useless efforts.

Prevention practitioners must continually do things to assure teachers and parents that an intervention will be an asset in their lives rather than a hindrance. For example, a therapist can find out from a teacher how the teacher wants an assignment to be completed, and can then help the student fulfill the teacher's expectation without the teacher's having to repeat the explanation to the student. Likewise, the therapist can find out from the teacher why a student failed science and tell the parent. This saves the parent from having to call the teacher and the teacher from having to find time to return the call. Once teachers, parents, and other adults who influence adolescents' lives experience genuine relief instead of further burden from cooperating with therapists, they will be more accessible and cooperative in the future. The goal is that they will eventually come to see the therapists' involvement as a gift.

Specific Intervention Strategies in the Schools

As discussed in Chapter 6, home-based family therapists working with adolescents and their families emphasize positive communication, behavioral monitoring, consistent feedback, and problem solving. The strategies detailed here illustrate what can be done in the context of the schools.

Positive Feedback and Rewards

Therapists should check how adolescents' notes are taken, how assignments are recorded, and how work is done. Besides providing acknowledgment for good habits, they can also give hints for establishing new habits.

Making contact with friends can also be an important part of the intervention. With an adolescent's permission, a worker can meet the adolescent's friends or include them in positive activities that the therapist and the adolescent are planning together. This may encourage friends to respect the adolescent's relationship with the therapist instead of putting it down. The adolescent is also much more likely to continue engaging in positive activities if his or her friends are involved.

Therapists can also change teachers' reactions to adolescents by alerting them to notice improvements. Leaving a message for a teacher, such as "I watched John finish his social studies packet and put it in his bookbag tonight. Watch to see if it is handed in tomorrow," can remind the teacher to acknowledge behavior that he or she might otherwise take for granted.

Being a Role Model

When a therapist pays attention to the school bell, makes sure an adolescent has a hall pass, asks permission before using a room, says "Please" and "Thank you" to secretaries, and asks permission of the appropriate authority before taking a student out of class, the adolescent will notice. It is important to let him or her see that the therapist has to "play by the rules," just as a student does. For example, even though the therapist might want to have an immediate meeting with a teacher, he or she may have to wait until the teacher's schedule permits, just as a student may have to.

Monitoring

A therapist cannot monitor all of an adolescent's activities, but schoolwork and behavior are relatively easy to monitor because of report cards and attendance records. As discussed above, consistent monitoring of school attendance, discipline records, homework completion, and grades on a weekly basis is most effective. The therapist can do this through weekly (1) phone calls to a contact person, such as a guidance counselor; (2) visits to the school and appointments with personnel; and (3) inquiries to the adolescent for specifics. This monitoring communicates several simultaneous messages. First, it indicates that a therapist truly values an adolescent and is genuinely interested in his or her life. Why else would an adult go to the trouble of providing consistent and careful attention?

Another message is that it is possible for adolescents to gain control over their lives by paying attention to the details. Often adolescents are unable to recount on which days of the week they were absent, but through discussing these details with therapists, they may experience a greater sense of control. Furthermore, discussions about what the adolescents did in school can easily be extended to include the consequences—both good and bad—that those actions brought. Adolescents can learn the natural contingencies of their actions, such as "Teachers give higher grades for neat work," and "Teachers are more likely to think you are paying attention if they see you looking at them in class."

Weekly Report Cards (see Figure 7.1) and the official quarterly report cards not only provide material to discuss each week in sessions as mentioned earlier, but they also provide relatively unbiased outcome measures for therapist feedback and accountability.

Advocacy

A family therapist can have a significant impact on how teachers and others think about an adolescent. This, in turn, can determine teachers' constructive involvement in the adolescent's life. For example, a worker who prepares a football coach for a new freshman candidate by saying, "He's nervous because he wants very much to make the team, and when he's nervous he puts on a very angry face," can prevent the coach from jumping to the conclusion that the student is uncoachable because he looks so angry. Or a worker can advocate on behalf of a student who engages in frequent outbursts in class by persuading the teacher that the outbursts are not directed against her: "I know she walks *into* your class every day resolved to keep quiet and do her work, so her outbursts are not because she's determined to bother you. They may result from her extreme sensitivity to 'putdowns' from other students." This can change a teacher's feelings toward a student from defensive to protective.

A therapist can also intervene in more concrete ways.

> For example, when the school's Child Study Team was hesitant to risk spending money on an expensive, out-of-district placement for a 16-year-old learning-disabled student because she was frequently truant from her public high school, her therapist approached them in the following way: "I've been in the home many times and believe that if a van picked her up every morning for a special education school, her attendance would be much better than it has been in the high school, where she cannot do the work. Her mother will make sure she gets in the van." Instead of giving up on the girl, this Child Study Team placed her in a private school for the learning-disabled.

A therapist's opinion may sometimes carry more weight than that of the adolescent or even the parents. Once again, however, it is very important for the therapist to encourage parents and other family members to become advocates for the teen. In order to protect confidentiality, the following case example is a composite of several cases, but it reflects recurring issues that family therapists face, strategies that they use in preventive interventions, and outcomes they achieve. Many youth like Kevin have been identified by the schools for our Early Secondary Intervention Program (ESIP) or our Targeted Family Intervention (TFI).

Case Example. Kevin Barnard, a 14-year-old African American honor roll student in eighth grade, was referred to a therapist after being suspended from school because of his regular involvement in fights so serious that injuries occurred. After one such fight, the police were called and he was removed from the building. Eventually he was excluded from regular school, placed on probation by the court, and assigned to an alternative school. Interestingly, his behavior just before the police removed him from school illustrated the conflicting demands in his life: He turned to the vice-principal, handed her a report he had done for his social studies class, and asked her to be sure to give this to his teacher. He was a high achiever who was also being reinforced for gang-related behavior.

Kevin's mother, Ms. Cross, was cooperative in attending brief meetings with the therapist. However, she routinely repeated that Kevin was grown up now, and that she could not keep meeting with the therapist about him because she had to take care of her other children. She had five children, of whom Kevin was the oldest; her youngest child was born a month after Kevin was taken into our program. She and Kevin communicated well, seemingly like peers. They both knew that she expected Kevin to be in charge of his life without much help from her.

Although Kevin behaved in a mature and responsible way by completing his homework and getting himself to school on time every morning, he still needed adult help. The alternative school principal, not accustomed to meeting the needs of college-bound students, had placed him in a curriculum far below his performance level. His mother refused to intercede for Kevin, citing her newborn infant and her lack of transportation. The role of advocate thus fell to the therapist, whose first concrete impact on Kevin's life was convincing the alternative school principal to place him in a more rigorous curriculum. At the end of the school year, the therapist again had to intercede by requesting that numerical instead of pass–fail grades be put on Kevin's report card. Although this was agreed to, the therapist had to monitor the situation closely, as it was many months before the school fulfilled this promise.

Although Kevin was not in the habit of getting help from anyone, the therapist provided him with a new experience. That is, when Kevin expressed wishes to her during sessions, she could help him attain his goals. During the summer after eighth grade, she helped him get a job, at which he performed very well. She also guided him through problem-solving steps that would enable him to stay safe and out of trouble with the police while walking to and from the bus for his job. The bus stop was in a rival gang's territory, and he was likely to encounter boys who wanted to hurt him in retaliation for his having previously hurt them or someone they hung out with.

Kevin's reputation was that he became "crazy" when he used his fists. He cultivated this reputation so that other boys would be less likely to "jump him." The counselor, a European American raised in a middle-class suburb, found out (to her surprise) that Ms. Cross was also happy that Kevin fought so furiously, because she believed that he would get badly hurt and even killed if he did not fight.

The therapist met Kevin in his home once a week for a 50-minute session. Almost every week, the therapist had occasion to inquire gently how Kevin resolved the conflict between his goal to stay out of trouble with the police and his goal to keep his reputation as a dangerous fighter. Together, Kevin and the therapist analyzed the antecedents and consequences of his regular confrontations. She also always asked about schoolwork and acknowledged his performance. They talked openly in the living room or kitchen. Ms. Cross sometimes joined them for a few minutes, just to listen. At these times, the therapist would summarize for her (and Kevin) the dilemma that they were discussing—for instance, "Kevin's started out high school very well and has gotten himself into college prep classes, but he's in danger of being suspended for fighting when he's jumped in the halls."

The therapist's persistence with Kevin and his mother was rewarded twice during Kevin's freshman year, when his mother became more involved in directing Kevin's life and substantially addressed his dilemma. First, she arranged for him to transfer to another school system and live with his paternal grandmother, Mrs. Barnard. Ms. Cross had kept in contact with Mrs. Barnard for the sake of the children, even though the older woman's son, Mr. Barnard, had been in jail in another state for several years. Second, when Kevin's reputation followed him to the new school system and older boys jumped out of a car to chase him into his grandmother's house one afternoon, Ms. Cross arranged for Kevin to live with a newly married male cousin who lived an hour away and to finish his school year there.

The therapist acknowledged and reinforced the mother's constructive involvement whenever the opportunity arose. Whenever she could, she also informed the paternal grandmother, and then the cousin and his wife, about the issues she and Kevin discussed. This exchange of information occurred rarely, however, because all of his caretakers worked long hours, and usually the counselor found him alone in his "adopted home" when she drove to him for their weekly visit.

The therapist was probably the only person who knew how very lonely Kevin was, and how much hard work it was for him to transfer from one school to another, to stay out of fights, and to maintain his honor roll status. They continued to analyze weekly the day-to-day events that challenged him, as well as his newly evolving ways to handle the confrontations and fear. In response to the therapist's consistent focus on the consequences of his actions, Kevin slowly moved from "hitting in order not to get hit," to refusing to be drawn into a fight but asserting verbally that "my younger brother can beat you," to simply not talking to anyone and going to the library during lunch, to discovering that he could indicate to previous enemies on the street that he was not going to fight by simply saying, "What's up?" as they passed.

Among the many rewards that the therapist experienced in working with Kevin was the inadvertent discovery, after 10 months of meeting weekly, of what motivated Kevin to sit at home alone and do his homework so perfectly every day. It turned out that every Friday night, Kevin's father phoned him from prison and grilled him about what grades he had received on homework and tests during the week. Mr. Barnard had been a college student when he was arrested, and he expected his son to get the education that he had not finished. Kevin cared very much about what his father thought about him, and dreaded the disapproval he would feel if he received a B or got into trouble. The therapist had had a hidden collaborator all along, and she had not known it.

After 1 year, the therapist moved to another state. Kevin was moved again in order to reunite the family—this time into his maternal grandmother and stepgrandfather's house back in his original school district, where two of his younger siblings were now living. Kevin continued to do honor roll work in college prep courses. Kevin's therapist's supervisor was notified one afternoon, however, that the school board was holding an expulsion hearing that evening for Kevin because he was always being "jumped" in school. The supervisor called the therapist out of state, and she called to bolster a very lonely, depressed, angry, and misunderstood Kevin. Meanwhile, the supervisor wrote the following letter to the members of the school board, with whom she had credibility after 3½ years of counseling high-risk students in their schools:

Dear Board of Education members:

I just learned this morning that the educational future of Mr. Kevin Barnard will be discussed tonight. I know how difficult your decisions are regarding students like Kevin. I am hopeful that some of our experiences with and observations of Kevin will be helpful as you are making your decision.

I am the licensed psychologist who personally supervised Ms. P.'s work with Kevin Barnard. Ms. P. and I met each week to discuss his counseling, and I reviewed audiotapes of Ms. P.'s work.

I understand that the high school has decided that it cannot educate Kevin in the building this semester. Our experience with Kevin, however, showed that he completed his homework and did well on his tests, no matter what else was going on in his life. He was clearly very strongly motivated to learn and to earn his high school diploma. His self-discipline and achievement in the realm of academics were extraordinary. Thus I hope a plan can be developed so that Kevin can complete his education, even if he cannot do so in the school building.

Kevin not only was one of the most academically accomplished youth in our counseling program, but he also utilized and benefited from counseling as much as or more than any other youth. Without violating confidentiality, I can testify that this very bright young man can problem-solve and think through life dilemmas at a level far beyond his age. He met with Ms. P. faithfully every week for more than 1 year. It was up to him to remember to be at home when she came for counseling sessions, and he reliably was there waiting for her. While in counseling, he developed effective strategies to cope with the academic and social difficulties of attending three schools in one year. Because he was able to use counseling for his benefit so well, I believe that he could do that again.

I appreciate how complex this situation must be for the school system. Kevin is a unique young man. I hope that my recollections are helpful in your deliberations. Please call me at _____ if you have any questions.

Respectfully,

_____

It turned out that no one had pointed out to the disciplinary principal that Kevin was doing exemplary schoolwork. In retrospect, the principal realized that Kevin probably needed his protection instead of his wrath. The school board decided to continue taking responsibility for Kevin's education, even though they did not want him back in their building. They arranged for him to enroll in a county school for the academically talented. The school system also recommended him for a Saturday enrichment program, in which he earned the "most improved" award.

Discussion. This outcome exemplifies an important goal of behavioral intervention—enabling a client to get enough reinforcement from the environment to maintain positive behaviors. This means that therapists must help clients find that environment. Even adults need personal recognition, inspiration, and tangible rewards to maintain excellence; adolescents need them even more.

DEVELOPING EFFECTIVE SCHOOL INTERVENTIONS IN YOUR OWN WORK

Family therapists may not have the opportunity to include comprehensive school-based intervention of the type we have described above in their practice because (1) children and adolescents from many different schools may be in treatment; (2) mandates may restrict treatment to family interventions; (3) existing caseloads may be overwhelming; and/ or (4) managed care does not reimburse for home or school visits. We would therefore like to summarize the ways in which the lessons we have learned from our school-based work can be applied by any practitioner.

Lesson 1: One Visit Is Worth a Thousand Phone Calls

The first lesson we have learned is that it is important to visit the school at least once. It is often very difficult to connect with teachers, guidance counselors, principals, and assistant principals on the phone, due to the nature of their jobs. A teacher, for example, cannot be expected to leave the classroom in the middle of academic instruction. Phone contact is even more complicated when working with adolescents in middle or high school, who typically have five to eight different teachers per day. In some schools, it is difficult to know whom to contact. Guidance counselors, for example, may be assigned by grade or by some other system to which the therapist is not privy. In some schools discipline referrals are handled by the principal; in others by an assistant principal or vice-principal; and in still others by a "dean of discipline." When faced with this vast array of individuals, it is best to begin by asking the family members whom they would recommend. Some parents are familiar with the hierarchy of their children's schools.

If the parents do not know whom to contact, ask the child. Arrange to meet the parent and the child at the school one morning, and have the child direct you to key individuals. This can be very empowering for some students, provided that they do not have to be seen with you by their peers.

If you have a release from the parents, another strategy might be to go to the principal's office and introduce yourself; give the names of the child and family members you are working with; and ask the principal to help provide you with information about this student or to introduce you to the best person on his or her staff for this purpose. Be sure to take the time to "join" with each school staff member (especially the secretaries) whom you meet or talk to.

Often a guidance counselor is assigned who will facilitate the process of your meeting a specific teacher with whom your client may be having a problem. Be sure to ask for the best method to reach this counselor and this teacher in the future. Some schools have voice mail numbers, fax numbers, or (in some cases) e-mail addresses for individual teachers. Find out when a teacher's free period or lunch period occurs; this may give you an opportunity to be introduced by the counselor or principal. If this is not possible, leave a note with your phone number or pager number and encourage the teacher to call. (You should be aware that many teachers may not have the time to return a call during the day.)

Parents can be given similar advice, especially when their children enter high school. Many parents who felt comfortable and competent when interacting with their children's elementary school feel overwhelmed by the "cast of thousands" who may be working with their children in middle or high school.

Lesson 2: Check with the School on a Child's Performance Even if the Child Is Not Referred by the School

Many cases are referred by agencies other than schools. The presenting problems may be non-school-related issues (juvenile delinquency, conduct disorder, court-related issues, etc.), and they may consume the initial focus of the family therapist. Even in these cases, however, it is important to obtain a release and contact the school in order to find out if an adolescent is still attending school and, if so, how he or she is doing. This is very important, particularly with high-risk adolescents, who are in even greater jeopardy of becoming involved in problem behaviors if they are truant or failing in school. School failure is one of the most important risk factors for these adolescents (Loeber, 1990). For example, adolescents are more likely to be lured "to the streets" and to develop substance abuse or conduct problems if they are doing poorly in school or if they drop out (Kandel & Davies, 1992). Anything that therapists can do to reverse the cycle of school failure will help adolescents to succeed in later life.

Lesson 3: Establish a Contact Person in Each School; This Will Make Your Job Easier

Family therapists with large caseloads may feel overwhelmed at the prospect of contacting schools. This often mirrors the sense that parents have of being overwhelmed. It is useful to check your caseload to see the schools in which your referrals tend to cluster. If you locate a specific school, attempt to establish a relationship with a contact person who can be of help to you in future cases to ease your entry and information gathering.

Some agencies have found it helpful to establish one person from their agency who becomes the "school liaison," or to designate a liaison for every two or three schools in an area. In other cases, a week spent by an administrator of a home-based family program making contact with the principals of the main schools in your catchment area will be invaluable in facilitating the contact of each family worker for each case. Many agencies have found that this is a very efficient approach, and it can operate at the highest level, connecting administrators in agencies with the most important administrators in the schools. This can relieve some of the burden for individual family workers, while maximizing the impact of a school intervention.

Lesson 4: Empower Parents to Go to the School; Do Not Do It All Yourself

If possible, empower parents to go with you in the process of connecting with the school. As they gain in confidence and skill, begin asking them to follow up. Remember that your goal is gradually to turn over the job to them. You will continue to monitor them until this transition is complete, but if you have done all of the school interventions, the parents will not advocate as effectively in future situations. This is particularly relevant for parents with a number of younger children.

There are some parents who have to overcome very negative reputations in schools. A teacher once greeted a parent in our program by saying, "You're Johnny's mother. Well, no wonder he's having trouble. I taught you in eighth grade, and you were just like him." As indicated in Chapter 2, if you encounter such a situation, you will need to work with the teacher and the parent so that they can renegotiate their relationship and the parent can be seen in a more positive way.

As stated earlier, some parents are so alienated from the school system that they frequently get very angry at parent–teacher conferences or Child Study Team meetings. If you have established a strong relationship with such parents, remember that it is often beneficial to help them role-play ways in which they can strongly advocate for a child without "going off" on teachers, counselors, and school officials.

It is also important to recall that children who become problems in school are frequently labeled. Many families whose members have experienced racism, oppression, and/or discrimination in the past may be very suspicious of the school system, and do not necessarily assume that the schools have their children's best interest at heart. To a certain extent, this vigilance and suspicion are justified. Again, many African American parents are aware that their children, particularly males, can experience the "fourth-grade failure syndrome" (Kunjufu, 1985) and are disproportionately placed in special education classes (Jones, 1988). Once family therapists understand such parents' concerns, they can act as a liaison between the family and the school and help the two to relate more effectively.

Lesson 5: Keep Hope Alive and Expectations Realistic

Many teachers, principals, therapists, and parents have very high expectations of rapid improvement from interventions. It is important for the family therapist to help teachers, school officials, and parents to recognize and acknowledge small gains, small behavior changes, or slight increases in grades, and to praise adolescents for these. The family therapist may have to reframe these gains and repeat them often to teachers and parents alike.

It is also helpful sometimes to predict that gains may be slow at first. The adults can then be reminded of this as the interventions proceed. Some teachers and parents expect F's to change to A's immediately; they may therefore miss the transitional steps from D's to C's and B's. Remember that, in such a case, you as the family worker are often the "container of hope" for the school, the family, and the adolescent, particularly early in an intervention.

CHAPTER 8

Community Interventions

with TAWN SMITH MORRIS

Many family therapists and workers who are effective in engaging and joining with clients and their families do not perceive a role for themselves in joining with the communities they serve. However, community entry and involvement are particularly important when clinicians are working in a minority community, as community members may be new to the process of family therapy and other mental health interventions, and some may be suspicious of the workers or skeptical about the efficacy of the interventions. This reaction may be especially pronounced if key administrators or staff members are of a different race or ethnic background from their clients.

Often the initial phases of community entry are accomplished by a program director or an administrator. These ties, however, must be nurtured over time if credibility is to be maintained. It would be a serious oversight for community outreach to be given short shrift in later years.

Credibility and trust are major issues in all communities, and they have particular salience in ethnic minority communities, especially those in the inner city. Many members of these communities perceive themselves as having been disempowered and exploited by a range of agencies. Therefore, workers and administrators who enter these communities should be prepared to answer many confrontational questions, such as "How are you different from all of the others?"

A portion of this chapter was adapted from Boyd-Franklin, Morris, and Bry (1997). Copyright 1997 by the American Psychological Association. Adapted by permission.

The failure of previous interventions is a familiar issue for the families served by family workers, but on a systemic level, it is a much broader concern in the communities. In every community, there is a "grapevine"—an informal communication channel by which important information is passed on to other members. If an agency has a bad reputation among community members, individual family workers may face an uphill battle in attempting to develop trust and join with the families and individuals they treat.

However daunting this may seem to family workers, the task of community entry and joining should not be the sole province of the program director and other administrators. Positive interactions or experience with clinicians can gradually change an agency's reputation in the community, and just as a negative reputation advances along the grapevine, so does a record of positive interactions and accomplishments.

COMMUNITY ENTRY

In designing or implementing service programs, program directors or planners must identify key community figures. Planners and directors who do not live in the community can and should be aided in the identification process by staff members who are community residents. Program directors, administrators, and family workers should also make systematic outreach to community-based organizations; school principals and superintendents; pastors of churches in the area; the local police chief and officers; local judges and court officials; administrators and workers in the local child welfare or child protective services, the welfare department, and the housing authority director; the head of probation and other probation officers; and local politicians. Attempts should also be made to connect with "grassroots" community members, such as parents who are active in the schools, school board members, and neighborhood or block leaders, who often have a wealth of helpful information and ideas for the implementation of programs. As Chapter 2 has demonstrated, the Black church historically has been one of the strongest institutions in the Black community (Billingsley, 1968, 1992; Boyd-Franklin, 1989; Comer & Hamilton-Lee, 1982; Hines & Boyd-Franklin, 1982). This is also true in Latino neighborhoods and many other communities. Ministers often serve multiple roles as spiritual leaders, counselors, and community and political activists. Programs often see results from this type of multisystemic outreach as problems arise in clients and families, and family workers can draw on the preexisting relationship established by others to obtain help from these resources.

Maintaining Community Outreach

Just as home-based treatment requires a commitment of time and energy, so too do community interventions. Because of the demands on individual family workers managing a challenging caseload, it is unrealistic to expect them also to carry the responsibility for community intervention.

Agencies and family service programs have chosen to handle the issues involved in community interventions in varying ways. Some have seen community connections as an important part of the program director's role; this can work well in smaller organizations. In larger agencies, where many programs are under one umbrella, individual project directors might handle this function. Some agencies employ a staff member dedicated to serving as a community liaison, which can be particularly helpful if this person lives in the community and has a history of relationships within the catchment area.

When budget constraints do not permit an agency to employ a staff member whose sole responsibility is community liaison, many agencies have adopted an effective strategy of dividing the liaison function among a number of administrators, family workers, and staff members. Individuals within the program can be assigned to one specific liaison responsibility— for example, to a school, church, or community agency; to a housing development, neighborhood, or community board; to a welfare, child welfare, or child protective agency; to a court; or to a police or probation department. The agency then develops an inter- and intra-agency resource list available for all staff members. In this way, family workers will have access to someone "in house" who is helpful in finding resources for a client or family. Regular intra-agency case conferences or staff meetings can bring these individuals together. This can also work quite well within the framework of the multisystems model as an interagency strategy. A regular multisystems meeting once a month to which the different agencies involved are invited can eliminate redundancy and contribute greatly to coordination of services, particularly with "multiproblem families."

Entry Issues for Workers of a Different Ethnic or Racial Background from the Community They Serve

Throughout this book, we have discussed joining issues for family workers in connecting with families. Just as the "use of self" is crucial in clinical situations, it is also essential in community entry and interventions. The abilities to be genuine, open, honest, and flexible are crucial characteristics in all of these situations. As highlighted in Chapter 2, it is essential that administrators, family workers, and office staff have training in cultural sensitivity that is experiential and gives helpful feedback on the effective use of self in different cultural situations. This might include the ability to acknowledge racial or cultural differences openly and non-defensively, and to discuss areas of common ground.

Once again, the caution not to personalize initial reactions or challenges is very important. Clinicians' taking the time to learn about the community, and asking community members to introduce them to others, can be very effective. Workers need to be especially sensitive when connecting with or entering a new community, particularly when community members are from a different racial, cultural, and/or socioeconomic group. Making an effort to connect personally with local community members and leaders can go a long way in building credibility in cross-racial or cross-cultural situations, particularly in the case of a White worker or administrator who enters a Black or Latino community. Not surprisingly, this same process can be relevant for an ethnic minority administrator or family worker who is entering a predominantly White community.

Entry Issues for Workers of the Same Background as Community Members

As has been emphasized, it is necessary that agencies include a number of family workers and administrators representative of the ethnic or racial groups of the communities they serve. Those who know the culture and language can enhance a program's effectiveness. Whenever possible, agency personnel should also include residents of the community. This can do a great deal to build a program's credibility and to increase participation rates. For this to occur, agencies must actively recruit such workers. Ethnic minority organizations and newsletters, as well as community-based newspapers, are often good places to start.

The issues for minority workers in agencies and organizations often mirror the concerns of clients. Many such workers report experiences of racism, discrimination, or subtle disrespect in the workplace. It will be very difficult for an agency or program to build credibility in an ethnic minority community if its own workers are poorly treated.

For family workers who are of the same ethnic background as their clients, working in their own communities has both advantages and disadvantages. The advantages include the opportunity to "give back" to youth and families in their communities, and to become role models by virtue of their dedication and training. This is often very empowering for minority workers and clients. In addition, the cultural sensitivity of minority workers may result in an easier initial joining with families and communities: The subtle cues as to how one should walk, talk, and use oneself in the entry process may be more instinctual for them.

These workers may also face unique challenges, however—both in their interaction with the broader community and in their efforts with particular families. Minority workers who live or worship in the community where they work may find the concepts of "therapeutic neutrality" and "rigid boundaries" to be inappropriate and counterproductive when they encounter clients at community events, at church on Sunday, in the supermarket, at playground, or at school activities for their own children. Even large urban ethnic minority communities may be very enmeshed and interconnected. Although this close connection with the community can greatly facilitate the work, it can sometimes be very draining and create boundary problems.

Ethnic minority family workers and program directors are often surprised to discover that the suspicion that many community members have about outside systems and agencies extends to them also. Workers and administrators should not be surprised when community members or client families test these workers to see whether they have "sold out" or "forgotten where they came from." It is very important for supervisors to be sensitive to these issues.

Utilizing Strengths

The traditional strengths of African American families have been well documented (Billingsley, 1968, 1992; Boyd-Franklin, 1989; Hill, 1972; Hines & Boyd-Franklin, 1982; McAdoo, 1981; McAdoo & McAdoo, 1985; Williams, 1987). The strong kinship bonds and extended family ties delineated in Chapter 2 still exist for many families. In some African American communities, however, the exodus of the middle class has stripped neighborhoods of their socioeconomic diversity, and the only families left may be the working poor and those living in abject poverty. Amidst such material desolation, the strengths in these communities are frequently invisible to outsiders.

Whereas in prior generations many African American communities functioned cohesively as large extended families with mutual responsibility for child rearing and discipline (a style epitomized in the African proverb "It takes a whole tribe to raise one child"), today fears of crime, drug trafficking, violence, and gangs have led many families to retreat inside their homes in an attempt to protect their children. This has resulted in isolation, emotional cutoff, and often hopelessness, helplessness, and despair. The parent and family support group intervention to be described next was designed to provide an opportunity for parents and families in a neighborhood to meet and share information, reduce social isolation, and empower themselves to address the issues threatening their children and their community.

Latino families also have many cultural strengths, as described in Chapter 2 (Comas-Díaz & Griffith, 1988; Garcia & Zea, 1997; Garcia-Preto, 1996). Similar to African American families, in Latino families, there are very strong kinship bonds and extended family ties. For some Latino families, the Spanish language serves a unifying function in the community. Some Latino families, however, have struggled with inter-generational language differences. For example, parents and grandparents may speak Spanish, while their children are bilingual, speaking Spanish at home and English at school. Religion and spirituality are also important strengths in Latino families. Both traditional churches and *espiritistas* and *santeras* help to provide healing and spiritual help.

SUPPORT GROUPS AS COMMUNITY INTERVENTIONS

This chapter presents a case study that describes the development of a community-based parent and family support group. It illustrates the process of running and establishing such a group, as well as many of the important community entry issues. Historically, family support programs have often included parent and family support groups (Weissbourd & Kagan, 1989). Telleen, Herzog, and Kilbane (1989) and Pizzo (1983, 1987) have found that such groups serve to decrease social isolation and reduce child-related stresses among participants. Within the last 15 years, the family support movement has gained recognition as a viable intervention throughout the United States (Kagan, Powell, Weissbourd, & Zigler, 1987; Weissbourd & Kagan, 1989; Zigler & Black, 1989). This is indeed fortunate, given current pressures to cut federal, state, and municipal funding for the social service programs that disproportionately serve poor inner-city families (Zigler & Black, 1989). Properly designed family support programs can empower communities to fulfill their own needs (Bronfenbrenner & Weiss, 1983; Zigler & Black, 1989).

The Development of a Parent and Family Support Group: A Case Study

This case demonstrates the role of a parent and family support group in the process of community entry and empowerment in a predominantly African American community. Our original intervention incorporated home-based family therapy and school-based programs. With the help of an African American colleague, we were introduced to a local, well-respected Baptist minister who greatly facilitated our community entry process. Through the minister, the family workers were introduced to several key members of the church and the community: the assistant pas-

tor and the pastor's administrative assistant; the head of the local housing authority (of a low-income housing project close to the church); concerned neighborhood parents; the principal of the local middle school;
and eventually the high school principal. Early in the process, however,
the minister and other community activists made it clear that they saw
the need to offer parents and other family members a forum to discuss
common dilemmas facing them in raising their children. We therefore
proposed a parent and family support group in addition to our other
interventions. Because of the key role extended family members under-
take in child rearing in the African American community, other family
members besides parents were included in this group. (The change in terminology from "parent" to "parent and family" support groups indicates this inclusion.) The idea of such a group was received enthusiasti-
cally by the initial group of community advisors.

Although we found that many families had been long-term residents
of the housing development (some having lived there for more than one
generation), they described a high degree of isolation. Adults tended to
go to work, come home, and stay inside. With the exception of a small
group of parents and family members who organized neighborhood
crime watches and ran the tenants' association, there was little interaction. For the most part, overburdened parents and relatives struggled
alone to handle rule setting at home, school problems, peer relationships, and increasing gang violence and drug use among children. Parents and family members also complained about the lack of activities for
adolescents. Although community-sponsored sports teams were available for boys, there was nothing comparable for girls.

The parents and relatives were not vague or indecisive. They were
very specific about their needs: explicit guidance in disciplining children;
assistance in addressing academic and behavioral problems at school;
and a way of fostering supportive contact among themselves—a request
that stressed the importance of support networks, in this case as a way
of enhancing the ability of parents and other adult extended family
members to perform the parental role. Monthly meetings for the parents
and family members would be held at a community room in one of the
housing developments.

Early Meetings

Parents and relatives supplied honest feedback about the challenges of
getting a support group started. The need for supervised activities for
children during the adults' meeting was mentioned. Another possible difficulty discussed was the perceived lack of continuity involved in services
provided by the graduate students who were part of this intervention;

group members would not trust an interchangeable series of people coming and going in their lives. Our team was composed of three family therapists, two Black and one White. Many parents and family members expressed initial concerns about the presence of a White family therapist. Her honesty, sincerity, and commitment were important in winning their trust. The seriousness of the group members' commitment was undeniable when a severe snowstorm did not keep them away from attending a planning meeting.

It was decided that the first parent and family support group meeting would focus on how parents and family members can influence adolescents' behavior. This meeting was poorly attended by group members—only one parent showed up to join the township's director of social services, the manager of the housing project, the middle school principal and one of the counselors from the school, the pastor's assistant, a doctoral student, and two of the family therapists.

Interest was accelerated greatly when a gang fight at the middle school resulted in the arrest of 12 boys (ages 12–14), who were subsequently jailed for periods ranging from 3 to 14 days. In order to be released from jail and placed on house arrest, the boys were required to attend an alternative school program at the church set up by the school district. They began mandatory attendance at groups organized by the church and focused on preventing violence and building self-esteem. The adults' meetings changed structurally to respond to this crisis: Attendance was mandated by the courts and probation department; meetings were increased from monthly to weekly; and the location was changed to the church.

The majority of the parents of the boys involved in the fight were single mothers. Although two were on public assistance, most were employed in diverse occupations. Two fathers also attended the meetings, and there were three grandmothers in the group. One grandmother wished to be included as a preventive measure, even though her grandson was not involved in the fight. This grandmother served as a resource for the group. Ten of the families were Black, one was Latino, and one was biracial. Ages of group members ranged from the mid-30s to 60s. Only a few families formally belonged to the church, but many considered the pastor an important advisor, community leader, and champion of their causes.

The focus of the group was modified to respond to the changed circumstances in light of the school incident in the following ways: (1) The consequences of the fight became the top priority; (2) the majority of group members would no longer be self-selected; (3) attendance would be mandatory; and (4) the geographical area was expanded beyond the original housing development to include an additional neighborhood.

The last modification gave rise to a new conflict. One of the underlying elements of the school fight was a neighborhood-versus-neighborhood gang dispute, which made the location of the meeting controversial. Since the church was located near one housing development, parents and family members from the other one felt uncomfortable going there, especially when accompanied by their boys. A centrally located social service agency was identified as "neutral territory" and became the third meeting place.

The two parents who had originally been involved in the planning of the group did not have children who took part in the fight; they found that the changed focus left little time to talk about their concerns. As a result, they stopped attending those meetings and helped to form a new group.

In keeping with the multisystems model (Boyd-Franklin, 1989), key figures involved in the fight and its aftermath—such as the superintendent of schools, the principal and guidance counselors from the middle school, and the head of the police department's juvenile division—were invited to early parent and family group meetings to assist in the exchange of information among parents and relatives, the courts, and the school.

Early meetings were characterized by parents' and family members' rage concerning the way police and school officials had handled the fight. The children had been removed from school in shackles and transported to a local jail, and the parents and relatives had not been notified about the incident for several hours. Group members were encouraged to discuss those angry feelings. Many refused to believe that their sons or grandsons were involved in gang activity, and were extremely suspicious of the accounts of the fight given by school officials. They resented what they viewed to be the punitive aspect of their court-mandated attendance at meetings, based on the children's alleged gang activity.

These were emotional meetings. Parents and relatives questioned the authorities about their methods for handling the fight and suggested that they were motivated by racism. The group members also objected because first-time offenders had been grouped with boys who had a history of violent behavior. Voices were raised, and tears of sorrow and frustration were shed over the perception that these children had been treated like criminals. Finally, the members raised the issue of the impact this event would have on the children's futures: Would they be labeled as "troublemakers" for the rest of their school experience?

After this incident, a number of heated sessions were held, with all of the parents and family members discussing issues of violence prevention and youth gang involvement. They discussed their fears of the escalation of fighting from fists, to knives, to guns. Many of the group members continued to deny that their boys were involved in gang activities. Others struggled with conflicts between cultural/familial messages that "you fight if someone else starts it" and the reality of the havoc wrought by violence in their community. Once they understood the mixed messages that they were sending, they were able to devise clear and consistent messages they could offer the youth.

Development of the Group

After a few meetings, an important shift occurred. One key parent, Cookie Boone, an assertive and charismatic woman, began to move beyond ventilating her feelings to focus on what actions needed to be taken. The process of Cookie's development was a metaphor for the group's development. Two of Cookie's three sons had been arrested after the fight. In spite of her own resentment, anger, and suspicion, Cookie believed that the group members could exercise a degree of control over the outcome of the crisis. This was the beginning of parents' and family members' taking ownership of the group. It was also the time when the parents and relatives truly started to trust the therapists, whose consistent weekly attendance at these meetings over the first few months was crucial. The therapists proved to the group members that they could tolerate listening to the members' anger and keep coming back. They communicated that they understood the members' anger as a demonstration of their love and protectiveness toward their sons and grandsons, as well as fears for them.

A reality-based focus on problem solving in the meetings assisted group members in understanding how the energy of their anger could be channeled constructively. Parents and family members were able to see both the smaller and larger pictures. They decided that they needed to be firsthand observers, and they agreed to attend the alternative school program on a rotating basis. They were fearful that unless they could ensure that accurate reports would get back to the school board about their children's participation, misinformation might be communicated (perhaps for political reasons) that would preclude the children from being reintegrated into the general school population. They exchanged information about their boys' behaviors during group meetings and shared ideas about how to handle problems. During one session, parents and relatives composed a letter to the presiding judge citing progress they had seen.

When the boys were taken off house arrest and placed on 6 months' probation, the meeting schedule was reduced to once every 2 weeks. Some parents and family members were still resistant and angry at this continuing intrusion into their lives. Attendance varied: Some group members attended every meeting, whereas others attended inconsis-tently. On the average, five to nine members attended each meeting. One parent unfortunately resumed drug use and dropped out of the group; her children were placed in foster care.

When the new school year started, some changes had occurred. A number of the boys had begun high school. Parents started intervening when they saw incidents occurring between the boys in the community. They even transported boys they recognized on the street to probation meetings. Moreover, Cookie Boone had gotten a job in the high school working with the security department. One of their own would be right there as an eyewitness, ensuring that no unreliable secondhand reports would go unchallenged.

The move to high school by the majority of the boys created greater fears among parents and family members about their ability to teach them the new rules of survival. The old rule that "you'd better not come home beat up" could be superseded by the never-ending cycle of retalia-tion (sometimes with weapons) set in motion by "beefs" between rival "posses" or gangs from more neighborhoods than they had encountered at the junior high school. Management of day-to-day school issues, such as attending parents' night, getting involved in choosing class schedules, signing up for the football team, and preparing for Child Study Team meetings for special education students, were still important topics.

Another nodal event occurred when Cookie began to work with the high school principal to resolve a disagreement that developed during the first 3 weeks of school. Before consulting the counselors, Cookie invited the principal to come to the support group; this led to a series of weekly meetings at the high school that included all of the boys from other rival neighborhood gangs who were involved in the disagreement, their parents and relatives, and the parents and family members in our group. These joint meetings resulted in a decision to make peace among the various neighborhood youth gangs—a milestone important enough to receive local newspaper coverage.

Discussion at meetings over the next several months centered around exchanging information about ongoing legal issues; grades; school problems, such as how to help the boys walk away from provoca-tion and avoid fights; and keeping one another updated about the activi-ties of the boys in the community. There was a growing sense among many parents and family members that the meetings were leading them to a position of greater influence within the larger community. Resis-tance still emerged, but the heated debate that resulted was constructive, although those few group members who saw such ongoing dialogue as "trashing the program" made their disapproval known.

Cookie and one of the grandmothers began to attend community meetings to discuss a recreation center to be built in the county. They told us that they believed they might now have a chance to influence where the center might be built, because people outside their neighborhoods were aware of what had happened with them and with the boys.

Ten months later, probation ended for all but the two boys who had prior police records. Mandatory attendance at meetings was now over. At a subsequent meeting, 7 of the 11 remaining members stated their intention to continue meeting. Future directions for the group were discussed. Group members wanted to communicate about their children and their everyday problems. They also wanted to plan workshops on such topics as conflict resolution within the family. When they were asked whether it would be acceptable to admit new group members, one parent remarked to universal agreement that it would be acceptable as long as the newcomers were willing to make a commitment to attending: "We don't want people to come in just for self-interest or when there's a trip or something. We want people with a commitment to the community." During one meeting, the group members and family therapists had a party to celebrate the passage into this new, voluntary phase.

Many of the parents and family members have increased their sense of agency and empowerment as a result of participation in the group. As Rappaport (1987) and others have suggested, this concept is multi-leveled and can apply to communities and organizations as well as to individuals. It will be important, therefore, to observe how the group continues to influence the larger community over time. It has led to an increased interest in such groups in the community, and plans are currently underway to expand the services offered.

Confidentiality in the Community

Issues of confidentiality may arise for clients or families who are part of an ongoing group or who meet together regularly or occasionally as part of a program. For example, in the case study above, we describe parent and family support groups that were established in accordance with a court-mandated intervention. When individuals or family members missed sessions, other members of the group offered to contact them. Our initial reaction was to discourage such offers because of confidentiality concerns. As we listened to the parents and family members, however, we were able to move closer to a model of a therapeutic/support group, and we encouraged parents and other family members to exchange phone numbers and to support each other outside of the sessions. This approach was developed from Boyd-Franklin's earlier work with therapeutic support groups for Black women (1987, 1991) and in multigenerational family support groups for caregivers of children with AIDS (Boyd-Franklin, Steiner, & Boland, 1995).

A confidentiality issue that frequently arises in home-based work occurs when the appearance of a family worker in the community alerts neighbors and others that the family is being visited by an outside agency. "Outsiders" are often viewed with distrust, particularly if community members, neighbors, or onlookers view them as representatives of welfare or child welfare agencies, police, or probation officers (Boyd-Franklin, 1989). This can be even more obvious to neighbors if the family worker is of a different racial or cultural group from that of most members of the community. A family worker may want to discuss with family members how they feel about the worker's coming to their home. If they express concern, the worker may want to arrange an office visit or a meeting at the school, a local church, or community center.

Another "community" aspect of the confidentiality question can occur during a home-based family therapy session when a friend, neighbor, community member, or extended family member visits the family. The family therapist should not make a unilateral decision to include or exclude this person. Instead, as suggested above, the therapist should greet the individual cordially and ask the parents (or parental figures) whether it is okay for this person to be a part of the discussion. If the parents agree to this, including the new individual may give the therapist a greater understanding of the family's support system.

Discussion: The Road to Family and Community Empowerment

The case study described above illustrates many of the components of a multisystems approach (Boyd-Franklin, 1989) and a family support model (Bronfenbrenner & Weiss, 1983; Kagan et al., 1987; Pizzo, 1987; Telleen et al., 1989; Weissbourd & Kagan, 1989; Zigler & Black, 1989). The first and most important of these is empowerment through community, parent, and family involvement. Small gains in self-determination should be recognized and acknowledged in the group. It is important that therapists become less directive and take on a more facilitative role as parents and family members demonstrate their empowerment. For instance, in the group just described, when Cookie invited the principal before consulting the group leaders, the facilitators supported this initiative and reframed her action as one of "taking charge" or empowerment. Therapists should not become involved in power struggles about control. A second key component, often present in work with minority parents, is helping them to channel their justifiable anger and rage about perceived racism and discrimination into constructive community action and activism. The case study also illustrates more general principles of community interventions that are helpful both to program administrators and to family workers.

PRINCIPLES OF COMMUNITY INTERVENTION

We conclude this chapter by summarizing 10 main principles of community intervention, based on our experience and that of others (e.g. Muñoz, Snowden, & Kelly, 1979).

• *Outreach.* Throughout this book, we have stressed the importance of outreach not only to clients and families, but also to the community in terms of key individuals and agencies.
• *Flexibility.* One of the most important aspects of community entry is the ability of the treatment providers to tolerate initial ambiguity and be flexible—or, as one of the parents in the group often stated, to "go with the flow." The ability to change direction and to create new avenues or opportunities when obstacles are encountered is critical. In the case just described, rigidity and unnecessary limits might have derailed the group creation process at any point. This issue is also related to empowerment. As parents take more leadership in the group process, therapists need to begin facilitating the process of transfer of ownership, responsibility, and power in the group to the parents and family members. Natural leadership inevitably emerges, and this should be encouraged so that the process of community support and empowerment can continue. This is also consistent with the next principle for therapists—cultural competency.
• *Cultural competency.* Boyd-Franklin (1989) and Boyd-Franklin, Aleman, Jean-Gilles, and Lewis (1995) have demonstrated that programs must be designed with particular ethnic/racial/cultural strengths in mind. The program described above utilized the role of the Black Church and its minister to help in the process of entry and community involvement. Consistent with African American cultural beliefs, the parent and family support process emerged partly from the perception of the self-defined needs of this community.
• *Credibility and commitment.* The case presented above is an excellent example of the process of building community trust and credibility. The family workers (as a Black–White team) and early counselors were openly challenged at first as to their role in the community. Parents and family members insisted that the group leaders establish credibility. It is important that therapists, particularly in cross-racial situations, see this challenge as an effort by parents and families to protect their com-

munity; it should not be taken personally by therapists, but should be addressed honestly and nondefensively as part of the therapeutic process. Program directors and family workers must recognize that this process is a gradual and unending one. Efforts to establish credibility should not be made once at the beginning of a program and then ignored in the subsequent years. Minority communities and families will often test therapists' commitment to staying involved, particularly when anger is expressed or when crises occur.

• *Community visibility.* In order for the credibility and trust described above to be established, it is important for agency representatives, both administrators and workers, to be "visible" in the community. This might involve participation in local events such as health fairs, school programs, and school board meetings. It might also include, particularly for program administrators, membership on community boards, coalitions, and partnerships. We have contributed in many of these ways in the different communities that we have served.

• *Focus.* Therapists must help to provide a clear problem-solving focus initially, because many families are so overwhelmed with problems that their anxiety can "flood" and engulf the group. A focus on positive problem solving and behavioral change for at-risk children and adolescents, and an emphasis on multisystems interventions in schools, community agencies, police, courts, and the juvenile justice system, are essential. A clear problem-solving approach can empower parents and families to effectively navigate the complex systems that affect their lives and those of their children.

Muñoz et al. (1979), in their excellent discussion of community-based research, also point out that so much of the process of building credibility in any community relates to the ability of agencies and workers to respond positively, actively, and decisively to unexpected events or opportunities. For example, in the case presented above, the family workers volunteered to begin a parent and family support group. This provided unexpected opportunities to demonstrate their commitment to the community and the important contributions of mental health workers in providing crisis intervention services.

• *Reciprocity.* Another key concept is the ability of a program to give back to the community. This may involve responding when community crises occur. Tragic community events (e.g., a homicide, suicide, or other major loss) or natural disasters (e.g., a storm, hurricane, flood, or fire) are opportunities to give something back and to be visible in terms of community service.

• *Responsiveness to community goals.* Muñoz et al. (1979) also discuss the ways in which the goals of the community members may differ from the program's goals. For a program to have continued viability, it is important that community members, including the clients and families served, perceive the agency and the workers as being responsive to the goals and needs of the community and the families. For example, in the case example above, the family workers had to adjust their goals when a community crisis led to the realization that gang violence prevention and positive after-school activities for youth were perceived as major needs of the community.

• *Negotiation of values.* Just as in the work with families and clients, community entry and interventions require a negotiation of values (Aponte, 1985, 1995; Boyd-Franklin, 1989) among the program, the administrators, the workers, the clients, families, and other community members. In the case example discussed above, there was negotiation among the parents/family members, the adolescents, and the family therapists. This was particularly apparent in the discussion of the messages the adults had given to the children with regard to the initiation of and responses to violence. Many of the group members reported that they cautioned their youth not to initiate violence, but sanctioned fighting if the youth were attacked first. The workers had to walk a very narrow line of validating these African American and Latino cultural beliefs, while helping the parents and relatives to see the dangers that might result now that guns had replaced fists. This frank, respectful dialogue and gradual negotiation of values between the clinicians and the families ultimately led to proactive community interventions.

• *Staying power and avoiding burnout.* These two concepts are presented together because of their close interrelationship. In order for programs, agencies, administrators, program directors, or family workers to have staying power and to avoid burnout, it is crucial that they receive support for their work, including the community-related aspects. Many programs and agencies do not recognize the central role of community entry and outreach in their overall mission. In these cases, administrators and workers who try to accomplish these interventions in addition to their "day jobs" quickly become overwhelmed and burn out.

Administrative support in terms of time for the interventions discussed in this chapter or "comp time" for evening meetings can go a long way in recognizing the importance of community outreach. Validation for administrators and workers who take on these challenges can prevent burnout and promote their staying power or longevity in their roles. The opportunity to receive training, supervision, and consultation on these community interventions can also become an antidote to the burnout of staff. (See Chapter 11.)

CHAPTER 9

A Multisystems Case Example

with NANCY BLOOM

Throughout this book, we have provided case examples that have illustrated particular aspects of our work. This chapter provides a comprehensive case illustrating many aspects of our approach to treatment: the multisystems model, including the roles of the school, court, police, child protective services, and residential treatment; the value of home-based family treatment; the process of joining as a way of getting past the "resistance" of an initially reluctant adolescent and family; and the value of community outreach.

DESCRIPTION OF THE FAMILY

Angela, an African American girl (age 14), and her family were referred for family intervention by her school guidance counselor. Her family was working-class, and a great deal of informal adoption (Boyd-Franklin, 1989) had occurred within the extended family. The immediate family at the time of referral consisted of Anna Taylor (a.k.a. "Aunt Anna"), who was 58 years old and the head of the household; her daughter, Carla (age 23); her nephew and legally adopted son, Jason (age 10); her niece, Angela (age 14); and Carla's son, Brian (age 7). (See Figure 9.1.) Angela had been living with this family for 2 years.

Ms. Taylor worked full time in a factory. Carla worked part-time in a grocery store. Ms. Taylor had never married Carla's father, and he was only peripherally involved in their lives. Jason, who was legally adopted

GENOGRAM

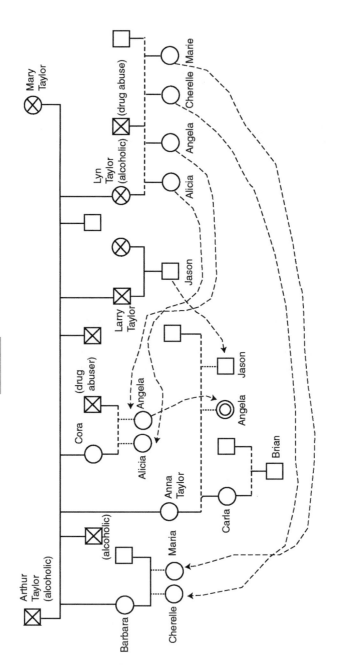

FIGURE 9.1. Genogram depicting Angela, her current immediate family, and her extended family. Dotted lines indicate patterns of informal or formal adoption of children within the extended family; dashed lines indicate individuals were unmarried; an X through an individual's symbol indicates a death.

164

by Ms. Taylor as a baby, was the son of Ms. Taylor's deceased brother, Larry. Jason, in fourth grade, was interested in baseball, while Brian, in second grade, enjoyed singing. Angela, an eighth-grader, enjoyed dancing, being with her friends, and "doing hair." She wanted to be a cosmetologist.

PRESENTING PROBLEMS

Angela was referred for treatment by her middle school guidance counselor. She was repeating eighth grade and was failing most of her classes. She was described as a behavior problem as well: During class she regularly got out of her seat, was disrespectful to teachers, and often talked out of turn to her peers. Moreover, the guidance counselor was concerned about the possibility of negative peer involvement, because Angela was involved in many altercations and fights with peers. She was very uncomfortable being the oldest girl in her class. The counselor also reported that Angela wanted to identify with older girls in the community rather than with her classmates. Many of these older girls had a history of behavior problems, and one had a substance use history. Finally, the counselor suggested that Angela did not accept responsibility for her actions.

Ms. Taylor complained that Angela wanted a lot of her attention and that she was jealous of Brian and Jason. Ms. Taylor also reported that Angela did not apply herself to her homework and/or chores, and that she often had to tell her more than once to do her work.

Angela complained that Ms. Taylor did not have enough time for her. She also reported that she did not get along with Jason and Brian, and that they were loud and noisy. In addition, Angela did not fully align herself with Ms. Taylor's Baptist religion. Although she sometimes liked going with her to church services, she suggested that it was too restrictive and time-consuming. Finally, Angela wanted to know more about her own nuclear family.

FAMILY HISTORY

Angela's biological mother, Lyn, had been the youngest of eight children. Lyn's mother, Mary, had died while in her 30s, leaving the eight siblings in the charge of 17-year-old Barbara, the oldest child. Ms. Taylor (Anna) and Cora were also Lyn's older sisters (see Figure 9.1). Lyn had a history of alcoholism. Angela reluctantly acknowledged that Lyn had often been intoxicated when at home and would disappear for hours to go to a local bar, leaving Angela and her siblings alone for long periods of time. (It was revealed later that during one of those times, at age 5, Angela was sexually abused by a male friend of her mother's.)

Lyn had had four children prior to her death in a car accident when she was 33 years old; she was driving while intoxicated at the time. After her death, all of her children were placed with extended family members. The firstborn was Alicia (now 15). She lived with Lyn's sister Cora, and both kept in close contact with Ms. Taylor. Angela, Lyn's second child, recalled that she and Alicia were "always together" as young children. Cherelle (now 12) and Marie (now 11) were born later. They lived with Barbara in North Carolina. Angela dreamed of visiting them soon.

With the exception of Angela, all of Lyn's children were permanently placed after their mother's death. Angela, however, had been in two homes. She was originally taken in by her Aunt Cora, where she lived with her sister Alicia for approximately 2 years. At age 12, Angela was sexually abused by a neighbor's son; the boy gave Angela alcohol and marijuana, and then molested her. This boy's mother was a close friend of Aunt Cora. When he was accused, this caused many problems in the household, and Angela was sent to live with Ms. Taylor.

The transition to Ms. Taylor's household was not easy for Angela. First of all, the composition of the family group was different from what she had been accustomed to. In addition, Angela was worried about Ms. Taylor's knowledge of the incident of sexual abuse and of her alcohol and marijuana use. She feared that Ms. Taylor "blamed" her and was waiting for her to "mess up." Angela also seemed to have difficulty sharing Ms. Taylor's attention. In addition, Ms. Taylor was stricter than Lyn had been; she raised her voice and used corporal punishment more freely than Angela had experienced prior to this time. Finally, Ms. Taylor's strict religious beliefs and traditions were uncomfortable for Angela, who had not been previously exposed to formal religious practices.

DESCRIPTIONS OF ANGELA, MS. TAYLOR, AND OTHER FAMILY MEMBERS

Angela presented as a needy young woman, craving attention from Ms. Taylor and other adults. She seemed to be hurt easily when not heard or criticized, and she appeared as depressed, angry, and/or agitated. She reported that she thought about her mom daily and missed her a great deal. Angela was pleasant and respectful toward the therapist. She was also thoughtful and quite capable of seeing another person's perspective. Angela reported that she was especially sensitive to loud noise and that

Ms. Taylor was "always yelling." She appeared older than her age and was well developed.

Ms. Taylor acted as caretaker for her extended family. She was quite protective of her children, both biological and informally adopted, and felt a strong love for all. Ms. Taylor was especially concerned that Angela would get involved in the wrong neighborhood crowd, and/or would "follow in her mother's footsteps" and use drugs and alcohol. She looked to her religion to help her in the children's upbringing. Although she was capable of communicating her thoughts and feelings well, Ms. Taylor, as a rule, did not do so with her children; she indicated that she expected her children to learn "how to read her." As a result, Angela was somewhat insecure in her relationship with Ms. Taylor. Because they did not "read" each other well, they did not understand each other's stance. Ms. Taylor appeared also to be lonely. Although she saw her sister Cora often, their conversations were superficial. According to her, both women kept their thoughts and feelings to themselves. Ms. Taylor could at times be very angry, rigid, and rejecting of Angela. At other times, she could be very supportive and loving toward her.

Carla presented as immature, wanting to be taken care of by her mother. She had few responsibilities in the house. Her son, Brian, was largely raised by her mother, Ms. Taylor. Although they were friendly children, Jason and Brian were extremely playful and often loud. Angela found their behavior very annoying.

CASE FORMULATION

Loss had significantly affected the members of this family. Throughout both sides of the extended family, there had been a tremendous loss of life at an early age. Angela's mother had lost her biological mother at about the same age that Angela then lost hers. Angela continued to experience loss as she moved from her Aunt Cora's home to Ms. Taylor's. It must not be forgotten that these losses had affected all members of the family and not just Angela. Angela's mother, Lyn, was the sister of Ms. Taylor and the aunt of Carla; therefore, they also experienced her loss. Angela, in particular, exhibited much difficulty as a result of the losses she had suffered. For example, she often appeared depressed; this exhibited itself in angry, agitated, and acting-out behavior—a reaction often observed as a response to sadness by children. Angela's unstable childhood could also partially account for her neediness. In response to her history of loss, Angela constantly sought the attention of Ms. Taylor and other adults in her life.

It seemed possible that Angela's poor academic performance might be related to her depression and neediness as well, because her teachers reported that Angela was intellectually capable of grasping the academic material. Angela's performance on standardized tests confirmed that she had more ability than she exhibited in school, and that her intellectual functioning was in the average range.

Since Ms. Taylor did not communicate in a direct fashion, her household rules and regulations were often not made clear to Angela; as a result, Angela was often unsure of what was expected of her. In addition, although Ms. Taylor apparently cared a great deal for Angela, Angela could not hear this message because Ms. Taylor presented it in so vague a fashion. In the same vein, Angela often misunderstood Ms. Taylor's playful teasing, misinterpreting her intent as negative.

A further problem for this family revolved around differences in emotional style. Because of her sensitivity to noise, Angela would physically shrink back from situations that were loud and obtrusive. Ms. Taylor yelled at the children a great deal. Angela became quite anxious when discussing the loud verbal reprimands.

Finally, Angela's mother's alcoholism and Angela's own history of sexual abuse—and Ms. Taylor's fears that she would become involved with drugs—became part of this family's projection process, resulting in Angela's scapegoated position.

MULTISYSTEMIC LEVELS OF INTERVENTION IN EARLY TREATMENT

Home-Based Family Intervention

In the home-based portion of the early interventions with this family, it was most important to join with Ms. Taylor. Until the family therapist could hear what she had to say, Ms. Taylor could not in turn hear Angela—which was, of course, what Angela desperately needed. As the family therapist validated her concerns, Ms. Taylor felt free to understand Angela's perspective, since she was no longer caught up in her own issues.

The family therapist regularly joined with all family members during home visits, greeting each person by name when she arrived. It was also important to join with Angela directly. She especially needed to hear the positive comments of the family therapist in the initial stages of treatment, so that she could feel good about her attempts at positive behavioral change. Early in their work together, Ms. Taylor had difficulty even seeing, much less rewarding, any improvements Angela made. As was the case with Ms. Taylor, joining with Angela allowed her to see and more readily understand Ms. Taylor's perspective. This led to better, more honest, and more forthright communication between the two.

It was important, too, that the worker reframed Ms. Taylor and Angela's statements toward each other. The reframe was not difficult to find, as Ms. Taylor and Angela had strong positive feelings for each other. The problem, rather, was in teaching each to communicate these sentiments. This was not an easy task, especially for Ms. Taylor.

Other goals of the home-based treatment included clarifying rules and expectations, as well as implementing a behavioral program to encourage prompt completion of chores and room cleaning for all of the children. It was also particularly important to be respectful of Ms. Taylor's religious beliefs, as they had a tremendous impact on the family's lifestyle.

A number of home-based sessions included the entire family. In one, a genogram (see Figure 9.1) was constructed with all family members present. This provided the therapist with an opportunity to explore the many deaths and other losses that Angela and her family had experienced. This was very difficult for the entire family, especially Angela. The death of her mother was initially too painful for her to discuss. The issue of loss was followed up in a number of subsequent family sessions. In one very moving session, Ms. Taylor shared with Angela how much she also missed Angela's mother, Lyn. She shared with Angela that when they were growing up, she had often helped to take care of Lyn, who was her youngest sister. With the therapist's help, they were able to hold each other and share their grief.

Different subsystems of the family were included in sessions when appropriate. The entire family (all of the children, Carla, and Ms. Taylor) were included in sessions such as the grief work described above and those in which plans for cleaning and chores were discussed. More often, the therapist worked with subsystems of the family; the most common grouping consisted of Ms. Taylor and Angela.

School Intervention

An important initial aspect of the school-based intervention was to talk with and listen to Angela's teachers. Receiving empathy from the family worker allowed the teachers to be more empathic toward Angela. Some, in response, went out of their way to help Angela, and in more than one instance they advocated for her. These teachers were able to see Angela's behavior from a different, perhaps less negative frame of reference.

Through connecting with the teachers on a regular basis, the family therapist was able to get regular information about Angela's school progress. In order to keep track of her homework assignments, Angela was given an assignment book to be signed on a daily basis by each of her classroom teachers. If all homework was completed and no demerits were incurred during a 2-week period, Angela was rewarded by spending more "private time" with Ms. Taylor. For example, they might go out for fast food after their treatment sessions.

By midsemester, it was clear that Angela was trying to complete and keep up with her school assignments. She often needed help with her homework, however, and Ms. Taylor reported that she did not have the time or patience to provide tutoring. The family therapist, through the school guidance counselor, was able to intervene and ask that Angela be enrolled in an after-school "homework club." Angela's grades by the end of the semester were C's, and she was no longer failing any classes. The family therapist worked with Ms. Taylor and with Angela's teachers to help them to see and acknowledge the improvement in Angela's grades. This work was particularly difficult for them, because she was not yet obtaining the A's and B's that they felt she was "capable of achieving." (This reaction is a very common one, as shown in Chapter 7. It is very important that therapists help parents and teachers to acknowledge small gains. Without this continued reinforcement, students often become discouraged.)

It was also important to empower Ms. Taylor to intervene effectively with her children's schools. In particular, she was often perceived as "passive–aggressive" and "difficult" by Angela's school. The family therapist worked with her to role-play her meetings with school counselors and facilitated the development of her relationship with the school.

Community, Peer, and Spiritual Interventions within Home-Based Treatment

This family was also known to a number of agencies in the community. Ms. Taylor's strategy for handling misbehavior by Angela and the other children initially involved "shopping" for help—a fairly common strategy in families with multiple problems. As a result, a number of outside agencies were involved, including child protective services. The family worker had to help Ms. Taylor to begin to see the home-based family intervention as the place to discuss these issues. It took Ms. Taylor some time to develop trust in the family worker and to "put all of her eggs in one basket."

Angela's peer group became more of a concern for Ms. Taylor toward the spring of the school year, when Angela and another girl were found with "wine coolers" in school and were suspended. The therapist worked with the family to discuss concerns about the use of alcohol. She helped Ms. Taylor to express her concerns to Angela and to set limits for her directly in family sessions. Angela had begun to spend more time cutting classes with friends in school and staying out with older friends after school. In one session, Ms. Taylor voiced her concerns about the negative reputation of these friends in the community. When Angela violated her curfew repeatedly, the therapist helped Ms. Taylor to talk with Angela about her concerns and to set a firm, consistent curfew with clear consequences. Eventually, Angela began to realize that she would lose her few privileges if she did not keep her word. The challenges for the therapist were (1) to help Ms. Taylor be consistent, and (2) to help her to impose the consequences (not going out with friends and no phone time with friends for the rest of the week) without a stream of angry statements.

Ms. Taylor's religious involvement in her Baptist faith and her participation in their local church also became a focus of treatment. Ms. Taylor had tried—as many inner-city African American parents and parental figures do—to protect the children, including Angela, from "the streets" by involving them in church activities. Ms. Taylor's strategy had been to fill up the children's after-school time with activities at the church. Angela did not object to the religious services and actually enjoyed the fellowship, but she resented the restrictions imposed upon her. In her attempts to keep Angela from being with the wrong crowd, Ms. Taylor had initially refused to allow her to have friends at the house or to interact with adolescents except for those affiliated with the church. With the family worker's help, Ms. Taylor was encouraged to allow the kids to have friends of whom she approved visit the house when she was at home, where they could talk and listen to music under her watchful eye. This was intended to give Ms. Taylor an opportunity to monitor the children's friendships.

There were a number of sessions in which Ms. Taylor was encouraged to talk to Angela and the other children about her spiritual beliefs and her hopes of protecting them from "the streets." In one very moving session, Ms. Taylor and Angela were encouraged to pray together in the session for the ability to understand each other better. This was a very powerful intervention: It reframed some of the more negative aspects of their interaction and helped to fuel the development of hope in the family.

Religious and spiritual interventions were particularly important with this family, in accordance with the salience of these beliefs in the Black community. It is quite common for highly religious parents and guardians to encounter major conflicts with adolescent children, who may perceive church and formal religion as extremely restricting.

Treatment Progress

The area of most improvement was in the home. Angela, in particular, seemed more content in her relationships with family members. She felt less isolated and more a part of the family. She reported that her cousins did not annoy her as they once did, and that she felt better listened to by Ms. Taylor. She also developed more empathy for Ms. Taylor's inability to spend a lot of time with her, due to other family and work obligations.

Angela appeared to have some secrets that she had not yet shared with anyone. Joining with Angela in a number of individual sessions gave the family therapist an opportunity to find out about her history of sexual abuse and to discuss these experiences. It appeared that during Angela's early years, her mother's parenting was inconsistent, and Angela and her sister Alicia were often left alone. Angela implied that "some things" had been done to her at age 5 by a male friend of her mother's, but she strongly resisted discussing these experiences—either by simply refusing to discuss them or by claiming not to remember them. After much persistence by the therapist, Angela was finally able, through drawing and discussing these issues in treatment, to begin to work through her own feelings about the sexual abuse. She had a great deal of anger at her mother for not being there to protect her, and at her Aunt Cora for "siding with" the neighbor's son instead of her when she was again sexually abused at age 12. After many months of individual work in this area, a number of very moving family sessions occurred, in which Angela was able to tell Ms. Taylor about these experiences and they were able to cry together. Ms. Taylor was able to hug Angela (a very rare occurrence) and offer her support. These sessions were a turning point in their relationship and in the treatment process.

Ms. Taylor also became better able to hear Angela's needs and to attempt to fulfill those needs. For example, although this was difficult for her to verbalize, she told Angela that she loved her and valued her as her daughter. This was important for Angela to hear, as she had heretofore believed that Ms. Taylor did not love her as much as she did the other children. In addition, Ms. Taylor started to acknowledge Angela's attempts at positive behavioral change. In the past, Angela's efforts had been obscured from her view by behaviors that were less than positive.

NEW MULTISYSTEMIC DEVELOPMENTS: THE PEER GROUP AND DRUG INVOLVEMENT

The improvement in Angela's behavior continued until the summer following eighth grade. At that time, Angela again became involved with several older girls in the community. She also again began violating Ms.

Taylor's curfew and coming in later and later. Things came to a head when Ms. Taylor found some "reefer" (marijuana) in one of Angela's pants pockets while doing the laundry. She confronted Angela, and a very angry shouting match ensued. The therapist received a crisis call, and a family session was held.

During the family session, Ms. Taylor was furious at Angela. She yelled, "How could you bring those drugs of the devil into my home?" She also told Angela that she was scared for her, and that she had been worried earlier because she had heard many rumors in the community about the drug involvement of Angela's friends.

As the summer progressed, Angela was on her own for hours while Ms. Taylor and Carla were at work. Attempts by Ms. Taylor and the therapist to find a summer program for Angela did not materialize. Angela became increasingly disrespectful toward Ms. Taylor. A number of interventions were employed. The family therapist met with Angela individually and in a session with her closest girlfriend to discuss concerns about her increasing drug and alcohol involvement. The goal of these sessions was to keep the lines of communication open. Angela was especially encouraged to verbalize her needs, feelings, and thoughts about her drug and alcohol use. Psychoeducational work was also done with her about the dangers of drug and alcohol involvement.

A number of family sessions were held to address family concerns about Angela's alcohol and drug use. Ms. Taylor was terrified that the younger kids would "follow her example." One important goal was for Ms. Taylor to make it clear to Angela that she was not to bring drugs or alcohol into the home. Ms. Taylor was also again helped to set a curfew for Angela and to establish consistent consequences. Firm consequences, including grounding (keeping her home), were instituted once more and appeared to work for a time. Furthermore, with the therapist's help and encouragement, Ms. Taylor contacted a friend of hers who was on the police force. He "kept an eye on Angela" and brought her home on a few occasions when she stayed out after curfew.

While limits were being set, another important goal of the family sessions was to help Ms. Taylor and the other family members to express their caring, worry, and support for Angela. This was hard for them to do initially, but it was even harder for Angela to hear. The therapist, in an attempt to move Angela out of the "scapegoated" position in the family (Minuchin, 1974; Minuchin & Fishman, 1981), also helped Ms. Taylor to have a number of general discussions with all of the children (not just Angela) about her concerns about drug and alcohol abuse in their community.

In mid-July, the situation worsened. On a number of occasions, Angela ran away from home and stayed overnight at her girlfriend's house. When she came home, Ms. Taylor said she "smelled of alcohol and reefer." One weekend night, Ms. Taylor was so frightened by and angry about this behavior that she called the police and had them take Angela to a local crisis intervention unit. As a result, Angela was hospitalized on a local inpatient adolescent psychiatric unit.

MULTISYSTEMIC CASE CONFERENCE

A drug screen on admission to the inpatient unit confirmed high levels of alcohol and marijuana in Angela's system. Once she was hospitalized, Angela's behavioral problems continued to escalate: She had a fight with another girl on the inpatient unit. The family therapist supported Ms. Taylor in requesting a multisystemic case conference. An eco-map was constructed (see Figure 9.2), and the key agencies that needed to be involved in the conference were clarified. The conference eventually included Ms. Taylor, the family therapist, the inpatient psychiatrist, a representative from the school system, and a worker from child protective services. After much debate, it was decided that Angela's increasing drug and alcohol involvement needed to be addressed. Those attending the conference recommended that Angela be placed in a structured residential treatment program for drug- and alcohol-involved adolescents.

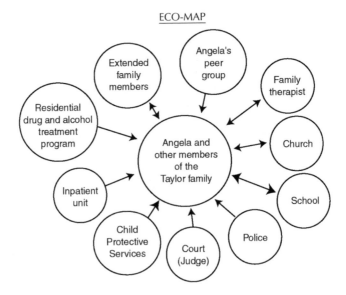

FIGURE 9.2. An eco-map showing all of the systems with which Angela and the Taylor family were involved. Arrowheads indicate directions of influence.

They also emphasized the need for a program that could address her history of sexual abuse. A decision was made to refer Angela to a residential drug treatment program for adolescents close to her home. At this residential center, she could receive appropriate educational programming and intensive therapeutic drug and alcohol treatment while in a safe, controlled environment. She could also maintain contact with her family, and family therapy would be provided.

Unfortunately, the recommendation for residential placement, even when supported by the local child protective and school systems (which would pay for this intervention), was only the beginning of a long, arduous journey. It was 3 months before Angela was actually placed in a residential setting appropriate to her needs, because so many efforts were required to move the process along. It took time for the local child protective services caseworker to gather relevant information about Angela from the various other agencies with which she had been involved, and even more time to put this information into the form of an application to treatment facilities. Angela's case then had to be reviewed by any number of staff members at each of the treatment facilities, who then had to come together, discuss the case, and decide whether to invite her for an interview. As it happened, Angela waited a month for an interview (originally a 2-month wait, but the family therapist intervened in the system to advance the interview), 3 more weeks for a decision about the acceptance, and 2 weeks further until a bed was available.

The plan set forth for Angela by Ms. Taylor, the family worker, and the other professionals attending the multisystemic case conference was almost sabotaged because of the length of the placement process. As noted earlier, Angela was "temporarily" placed on an inpatient psychiatric unit for those in need of acute care. The hospital vehemently protested Angela's lengthy stay, appealing to the court system for help to have her discharged. Although the judge seemed truly concerned that Angela's placement should meet her needs (he spoke at length with the family worker on a number of occasions), the court could no longer require the hospital to be responsible for Angela. It finally gave child protective services 2 weeks to place her. Unfortunately, placement at an appropriate residential adolescent drug and alcohol treatment program had not yet been offered to Angela; therefore, she was moved to and subsequently placed in a group home. This program offered psychotherapy only once a week, and it provided no drug or alcohol treatment or any work for survivors of sexual abuse. This placement was not acceptable to either Ms. Taylor or the family therapist, but once it was completed, the officials at child protective services felt that their responsibility was fulfilled, even if their recommendations had not been followed.

A week after Angela was placed by court order, a facility that could meet all of Angela's special needs offered her a placement. Child protective service officials stated that changing placements was not possible, and they were not receptive to moving Angela. The family therapist and Ms. Taylor worked as a team so as not to lose the opportunity to place Angela in this treatment program. Together, they contacted the judge and asked that he mandate the plan that had been originally agreed upon. They also spoke with a representative from the multisystems case conference, asking that child protective services be contacted and that the recommendations made by the team be reiterated. In addition, they took turns calling the caseworker from child protective services, continually appealing for her help. Finally, the family therapist spoke frequently to the residential program that had offered the placement, assuring them that both Ms. Taylor and the family worker wanted Angela to attend this program. In the end, they were successful in getting Angela transferred to the residential adolescent drug and alcohol treatment program, which also had a special program for victims of sexual abuse.

DISCUSSION

This family's experience illustrates the multisystemic complexity of many of the families seen by family workers. The family therapist had to work closely with the family members as well as with numerous outside agencies, including the school, child protective services, the staff of the inpatient unit, the police, the courts, and the residential treatment program. In order to empower Ms. Taylor and the family, a multisystemic case conference was necessary to bring the parties together.

Family therapists often encounter cases in which children's behavior escalates in the community and it is necessary to move to placement outside the home. The difference in this case was that because of the home-based family intervention and the growing bond among the family therapist, Ms. Taylor, Angela, and the other children, the family members were able to commit themselves to ongoing involvement with Angela and her treatment process. This would continue while she received intensive treatment in a residential treatment center. Too often in these cases, a cutoff occurs between the family and the adolescent. The combination of intensive multisystemic intervention and home-based treatment facilitated familial relationship building and helped to avoid this pitfall.

This case illustrates another very important lesson. Many family workers have, as their programs mandate, the job of family preservation. In many of these cases, the decision to place a child outside the home is seen as a "failure." This is unfortunate, because there are some situations—particularly cases of adolescent drug and alcohol abuse—in which residential treatment is in the best interest of both the child and the family. The family therapist in this case had the ultimate goal of family preservation and reunification. In the interim, however, Angela needed a residential treatment facility where she could receive intensive drug and alcohol treatment, as well as treatment and programming for her sexual abuse history, in a safe, protective environment.

The therapist also empowered the family to advocate for the residential treatment that would be best suited to Angela's needs. When this type of placement occurs, a family therapist can have a major impact by empowering the family to navigate the complex multisystemic bureaucracy involved; by preserving the family's contact with the child while in residential placement; and by continuing regular sessions of the family intervention before, during, and after placement, to ensure that family connections and bonds are maintained. In order to help Angela's family through this difficult transition, the family therapist attended a number of initial family therapy sessions at the residential treatment program and gradually transferred Angela and her family to the care of therapists in this program.

PART IV

RESEARCH AND SUPERVISION

CHAPTER 10

Research Evidence
for Home-Based, School,
and Community Interventions

with CAROL SLECHTA

Proactive family interventions enjoy solid empirical support. The intervention studies reported in this chapter all include components of outreach, be they home visits, school visits, or community interventions. Most have taken a multisystemic perspective, targeting the multiple influences in a child's or family's life. Although the effectiveness of specific intervention components cannot always be identified, these studies suggest that proactive, multisystemic interventions are more effective than "service as usual" with at-risk children and families.

Also of great importance to all family practitioners is the research on family risk and protective factors—that is, factors that have been found to heighten children's risk for academic failure, behavior problems, and substance abuse, and factors that have been found to protect against such risk (Bry, 1996; Bry et al., 1982; Smith, Lizotte, Thornberry, & Kroh, 1995). Indeed, it was these scientific findings that first propelled practitioners proactively out of their consulting rooms and into their clients' homes. This chapter presents an overview of family protective and risk factors, followed by a review of the characteristics and components of family interventions that have been found to be effective in reducing risk factors and enhancing protective factors.

PROTECTIVE PARENTING PRACTICES

Parenting practices that appear to reduce child and adolescent problems fall into two general groups: those predominantly taking place in the home and within the family, and those that involve contact with outside institutions. Protective parenting within the home involves the establishment of "close," or mutually reinforcing, parent–child relationships and positive methods of behavioral influence. Protective parenting outside the home involves monitoring and supervising of children's activities and relationships, becoming proactively involved in children's activities outside the home, and seeking necessary parenting resources (e.g., adult collaboration, day care, or information about normative developmental expectations for children). With these research findings in mind, family workers can proceed with confidence in encouraging these protective parenting practices in their treatment approach.

Maintaining Mutually Reinforcing Parent–Child Relationships

Evidence suggests that parents have more influence upon their children's behavior if the parent–child relationship has consistently been characterized as warm, intimate, nurturing, and nonconflictual. This protective effect apparently holds true across socioeconomic, ethnic, and racial groups, and for children, adolescents, and young adults. Parents whose children report close relationships with them are more likely to comfort children when they are afraid, have mutual communication between parent and child, center their attention on the child, and give children some choice or say in what happens to them (Brook, 1993; Johnson & Pandina, 1991; Kandel, Kessler, & Margulies, 1978; Streit & Oliver, 1972).

Brook and colleagues (Brook, 1993; Brook, Brook, Gordon, Whiteman, & Cohen, 1990; Brook, Whiteman, Gordon, & Brook, 1984) have studied the connections between children's behavior and parent–child relationships for 20 years—longitudinally and cross-sectionally; with mothers and fathers; in the middle class and the poor; and in Whites, Blacks, and Puerto Ricans. Defining attachment as "an affectional bond between parent and child that is long lasting and of considerable intensity" (Brook, 1993, p. 82), Brook finds evidence that strong attachment is protective. It heightens the effect of parental reinforcement of the child's conventional behavior, increases a child's emulation of parental behavior, and increases the chances that a child will choose friends whose values are similar to the parent's. In an East Harlem study of Black and Puerto Rican 7th- to 10th-graders, Brook (1993) also found that the effects of risk factors, such as having friends who used alcohol and marijuana, were offset by close mutual attachments between parents and children. Among 10-year-old White boys from the northwestern United States, parental acceptance correlated negatively with behavior problems in middle childhood (Dishion, Reid, & Patterson, 1988). An inverse relationship between family bonding and drug use initiation holds true across all racial and ethnic groups studied (Catalano et al., 1993; Stephens, 1996).

As adolescents mature, family closeness becomes even more important in protecting against problems. Family closeness appears to have its largest preventive effects in countering the influence of antisocial peers in middle and late adolescence (Duncan, Duncan, & Hops, 1994; Farrell & White, 1998). There is also convincing evidence that the influence of parent–child relations extends into adulthood. In a longitudinal study of adolescents who were heavy drug users, perceived parental warmth was found to be one of the most important variables that differentiated young adults (25–31 years old) who stopped using heavily from those whose heavy adolescent use continued right into adulthood (Bennett, 1995), with all the accompanying work-related, marital, and legal problems.

Family therapists, however, must guard against presupposing what makes relationships reinforcing, since important values vary across cultures. For example, mutually reinforcing relationships between Haitian parents and their children may not appear close to southern Europeans, because respect is more important in Haitian culture than sharing secrets is (Thomas, 1995). In addition, protective relationships are not limited to biological parents; there is ample evidence from Werner's (1989) well-known longitudinal study on the Hawaiian island of Kauai that a long-term, caring relationship with a relative or neighbor can be protective if a parent is unavailable. Throughout this book, we have given many case examples in which a grandparent or another relative has taken over child-rearing responsibilities when a parent has been unable to fulfill these. Such a person can also provide other protective factors.

Employing Consistently Positive Methods of Behavioral Influence

Positive parental behaviors have been identified and shown to be strikingly consistent across age groups throughout childhood and adolescence, and across demographic groups. These are specific parenting practices that family therapists will want to encourage. Positive parenting methods include clearly communicated expectations, rules, and consequences for misbehavior; ample praise and encouragement from parents for moment-to-moment compliance; and, when rules are broken, automatic, unemotional application of predetermined consequences. Typified by consistent reinforcement for socially adaptive behavior, positive parenting produces socially competent children, who are less vulnerable to problems. The broad effects of positive parenting are twofold: A child's positive behavior is fostered, and the parents develop influence that allows them to discourage potentially problematic behaviors as they occur.

Protection against early childhood problems is associated with well-established, enforced rules and standards of conduct; a predictable home environment; high expectations; encouragement to do one's best; and appreciation for efforts and accomplishments during early childhood. It has been found that parents who do these things when their children are 3–6 years old reduce the likelihood that their children will use marijuana and hard drugs (hallucinogens and cocaine) by age 14 (Block, Block, & Keyes, 1988).

The relationship between parental behavior management techniques and substance use appears invariant across ethnic groups. Catalano et al. (1993) examined the relationship between behavior management techniques and fifth-graders' problems in Black and White families. In both groups, what the researchers called "proactive family management practices" (p. 810), such as monitoring, praise, clear rules, and the absence of unfair criticism, inhibited elementary school students from experiencing academic failure, discipline problems, and drug use. No difference was found in the relationship between parenting style and substance use between White and Hispanic families of 9- to 17-year-olds. Nonusers' parents often had rules about homework, television, curfew, and drug and alcohol use. These "parents maintain[ed] control by clarifying appropriate behaviors, reinforcing them with praise and encouragement, and maintaining warm, caring relationships so that their children desire[d] to please and emulate them" (p. 480).

Parental reactions to individual episodes of problem behaviors seem to affect the probability that they will continue. If parents apply previously understood sanctions, such as revoking driving privileges, continued problems are less likely (Bailey, Flewelling, & Rachal, 1992; Christiansen, Goldman, & Brown, 1985; Kaplan & Johnson, 1992).

Parents who use consistently positive methods of social influence foster socially competent modes of interaction in their children; in contrast, aggressive and anxious modes of interacting are known to predict future problems (Kellam, Brown, Rubin, & Ensminger, 1983; Lindahl, 1998). Many families referred for help display the latter modes. Analyses of mother–child control exchanges in early childhood ($2\frac{1}{2}$–$6\frac{1}{2}$ years) reveal some apparently paradoxical findings about effective parenting techniques (Dumas, LaFreniere, & Serketich, 1995). Mothers of socially competent children actually initiate fewer attempts to control, and so do their children. These mothers' control attempts (commands, requests, or instructions) are reliably more positive, consisting of laughter, helping, approving, and expressions of affection.

Interestingly, effective mothers comply with their children's control attempts as much or more (almost 50%) than other mothers (35% or 20%); unlike less effective mothers, however, they respond very differently to the children's noncoercive attempts to control than they do to coercive (repeated) attempts to control. These effective mothers comply with 80% of their children's noncoercive control attempts, while actively refusing to comply with half of all coercive control attempts. Through their consistent responses, effective mothers actively train their children to influence others through single, positive requests. Less effective mothers (those whose children are less socially competent) do not discriminate as effectively between positive and coercive control efforts on the part of their children. They may never actively refuse to comply with coercive attempts, may comply indiscriminately to positive or coercive attempts, or may comply more often to coercive attempts than to positive attempts. In this way, they inadvertently train their children to use coercive means of social influence. Thus, paradoxically, parents who are less controlling and more responsive to positive behavior actually gain more short- and long-term influence over their children's behavior than do parents who emphasize control and who resist their children's positive attempts at social influence. Family therapists can share this paradox with clients, and thus can help them gain more influence over their children through loosening coercive control.

Evidence that these parenting methods indeed differentiate between families with problems and families without problems has been found for preadolescents (Dishion et al., 1988) and young adolescents (Greene & Bry, 1991; Krinsley & Bry, 1992). Microanalyses of interactions in families of children with problems reveal inconsistent, largely ineffective parental responses. These parents inadvertently provide "payoffs" for aversive behavior through positive outcomes (e.g., talking, attention, and compliance with coercive demands) and through the removal of aversive stimuli (e.g., allowing children to refuse requests). Although these parents are also observed to threaten, scold, and lecture their children at higher rates than do other parents, many of these reactions do not follow inappropriate behavior, and their threats may not be carried out. In addition, they do not routinely reinforce desirable behavior with praise and support. Patterson (1995), who has performed extensive studies of family interactions, portrays the outcome of this process as children become older and parents lose control of their adolescents' behavior. "For example, parents become increasingly hesitant to pressure children to tell [parents] where they are going or what they are doing. The parents know that even if they had the information, they would be unlikely to win in a discipline confrontation involving any of these issues" (p. 95).

Monitoring and Supervision

Evidence is accumulating for both direct and indirect protective effects, across demographic groups and developmental stages, of parents' knowing where and with whom their children spend time. There is strong evidence, for instance, that parental surveillance has a direct effect on whether or not drugs and alcohol are sampled in middle childhood. This knowledge is critical, since it is well documented that the earlier substances (including tobacco) are used, the greater the chances of eventual substance abuse (Brunswick, Messeri, & Titus, 1992; Kandel & Davies, 1992; Robins & Przybeck, 1985; Smith & Fogg, 1978). Chilcoat, Dishion, and Anthony (1995) found that when urban, minority parents decreased their level of surveillance over 8- to 10-year-olds, the chances increased that the children would initiate substance use within 1 year. Parental supervision decreases 10-year-olds' substance use by reducing the time spent with deviant peers, with whom 89% of substance use begins (Dishion et al., 1988). Black parents who decided which friends their elementary children could see significantly lowered the chances that their offspring would ever abuse substances (Catalano et al., 1992). Furthermore, there is evidence that *each episode* of substance use is individually affected by expectations regarding that particular use. As mentioned above, even regular users (those who use 5–7 days a week) do not use available substances on days when they expect to "get caught" and be penalized by police or their parents (Beier, 1990).

Contrary to some popular assumptions, parental monitoring seems to become even more important during adolescence. In fact, there is evidence that monitoring is the primary deterrent to behavior problems in adolescence (Dishion et al., 1988; Forehand, Miller, Dutra, & Chance, 1997). This relationship was found for White 7th- and 10th-graders of middle and higher socioeconomic statuses in the northwestern United States (Dishion et al., 1988); for predominantly White and Latino 8th-graders (Richardson et al., 1989) and 12th-graders from the lower to upper classes in southern California (Stice et al., 1998); for Canadian White high schoolers from rural and small town settings (Smart & Gray, 1979); and for Black, poor 16- and 17-year-olds in Chicago (Ensminger, 1990).

Finally, the impact of supervision appears to continue right into adulthood. Young adults in more structured environments, such as the military and universities, report significantly less deviant behavior than do 18- to 25-year-old men in full-time jobs (Newcomb, 1988). In fact, throughout adulthood, there appears to be more antisocial behavior in occupations with less immediate supervision (Slattery, Alderson, & Bryant, 1986). Thus the first change that family therapists may want to help parents implement in their families is increasing family members' knowledge of the whereabouts of other members.

Being Involved with and Advocating for Children Outside of the Home

Research points to the importance of parents' involvement in their children's activities outside the family. Helping children meet and get to know friends is protective. Children's participation in conventional clubs, hobbies, and sports outside the home is likewise protective (Jessor & Jessor, 1977; Swisher & Hu, 1983). Often parents must first advocate for their children to get them enrolled in such activities, and then the parents must attend the activities with their children to keep them involved. Krohn and Thornberry (1993) found that the parents of 14- and 15-year-old northwestern U.S. city youth who did not have problems were significantly more likely to attend school sports events and religious activities with their children, whereas the parents of youth with problems were much less involved in these social networks. Going to a child's school for "back-to-school night" is clearly associated with better school performance (Dornbusch, Ritter, Liederman, Roberts, & Fraleigh, 1987). Adolescents whose parents help introduce them to the world of work show increased interest in its intrinsic pleasures, rather than disillusionment and cynicism, as they grow into young adults (Cotton & Bynum, 1995).

The evidence suggests that attendance at religious activities protects against many problems, both while parents are taking their children (Kandel & Davies, 1992), and in early adulthood after the family members no longer attend together (Brunswick et al., 1992). It is not known why parent–child religious attendance is protective; it may increase time spent together, reinforce commitment to conventional values and institutions, or provide a spiritual experience that competes with the thrill of getting into trouble. Religious practice may also have its effect by placing family members in a relatively trouble-free context among other people who support participation in constructive activities.

Seeking Information and Social Support

The basic requirements of protective parenting have been shown to be (1) warm, nurturant relationships; (2) positive behavioral influence; (3) routine monitoring and support; and (4) involvement in children's outside activities. These requirements, however, have become increasingly difficult to meet as changes in technology, housing patterns, and family mobility have stripped parents of traditional child-rearing supports—extended family members and lifelong neighbors. Meanwhile, the stunning growth of global communication and transportation increases the temptations, challenges, and demands faced by our children.

Today, even so-called "traditional" families—two parents, one full-time at home—can lack the necessary information, patience, and time to protect their children. The majority of families today, with two working parents or a single parent, find it extremely difficult to provide all of the protective factors. Depression, bereavement, health problems, and other psychological distress, which most parents experience at one time or another, disrupt necessary attentional, affectional, and monitoring skills (Dumas, Gibson, & Albin, 1989). For the most vulnerable groups in our society, conditions may be overwhelming. Poverty and its accompanying daily hassles can exhaust parents' meager resources (Belle, 1990; Parece, 1997). Drug-trafficking neighborhoods provide multiple reinforcements for children's involvement in illegal activities, defeating parents' efforts to counter their negative influence (Dembo, Blount, Schmeidler, & Burgos, 1986).

Increasing evidence suggests that proactive parents—those who actively seek child-rearing information and support—are able to counter these effects and reduce the risk of problems with their children. Low-income Latina and Black adolescent mothers who were responsive to and sought out support and guidance from adults who were not their parents, experienced lower levels of disruptive depression and anxiety while caring for their infants, even though their lives contained as much objective stress as those of young, mentorless mothers, who suffered more distress and anxiety (Rhodes, Contreras, & Mangelsdorf, 1994; Rhodes, Ebert, & Fischer, 1992). In a middle-class sample, Crockenberg (1981) found that the level of social support received and sought by mothers of 3-month-old infants related positively to the security of the children's attachment at 1 year. Social support for the mothers was most beneficial for the most irritable infants.

Further evidence that the willingness to seek and accept information and support can bolster effective parenting comes from a study of wives of men with untreated alcohol problems, who were parents of 3- to 6-year-old boys. After the men were convicted of driving under the influence of liquor, the parents were invited to participate in a program "to improve parent–child communication patterns." The mothers who took the most advantage of the program, attended the most sessions, completed assignments outside the sessions, discussed the most problems, and asked for the most help during the sessions benefited their boys' behavior the most (Nye, Zucker, & Fitzgerald, 1995). Women who share troubles with a confidante or circle of friends, and who receive emotional and/or instrumental aid, are less likely to become overwhelmed to the point that parenting is disrupted (Stack, 1974).

RISKY PARENTING PRACTICES

Neglecting Children

Parental rejection, underresponsiveness to a child's behavior, and underconcern about a child's well-being, at any time from birth to adulthood, seem to predispose a child to behavioral and emotional problems. From preschool onward, pressuring a child to "perform" while giving no acknowledgment or appreciation, also seems to heighten risk (Block et al., 1988; Shedler & Block, 1990). It is assumed that such parenting increases vulnerability to problems because the lack of emotional connection leaves the child unreceptive to adult disapproval.

If children do not learn to expect positive interactions with the first important figures in their lives, they may become immune to positive social influence altogether. Indeed, Allen, Leadbeater, and Aber (1994) found that among White, Black, and Hispanic 15- to 18-year-olds from three large cities in the northeastern United States, negative expectations in social interactions predicted increased delinquent acts in the next 6 months. Many studies have shown which conditions increase the likelihood of neglectful parenting: adolescent pregnancy (Furstenberg, Brooks-Gunn, & Morgan, 1987), unplanned pregnancy, poverty (Hendin, Pollinger, Ulman, & Carr, 1981), absent or stressful social networks (Dumas & Wahler, 1983), and parental depression (Patterson & Forgatch, 1990). Amelioration of any of these predisposing conditions reduces the likelihood of neglectful parenting and related behavior problems in offspring. Consequently, home-based family therapists often address parents' environmental stressors, social supports, and emotional problems in their efforts to reduce children's problems.

Abusing Children Physically or Sexually, or Exposing Them to Violence against Others

One of the riskiest factors in parent–child relationships is physical and/ or sexual abuse. In general, sexual assault raises the likelihood that significant problems will develop within 1 year of the assault (Burnam et al., 1988). Research during the past decade has revealed that both physical and sexual abuse are strongly connected with later emotional and behavioral problems (Clayton, 1992). Evidence suggests that both physical and sexual abuse, particularly in childhood, increase vulnerability to substance abuse two- to fourfold (Office of Technology Assessment, 1990; Polusny & Follette, 1995).

Some forms of abuse are especially destructive. Among male and females in detention centers, the more modes of childhood physical abuse (being beaten with hands or feet, being hit with a hard object, being shot with a gun or injured with a knife, etc.), the greater the severity of the individuals' crimes (Dembo et al., 1989; Dembo, Williams, Wothke, Schmeidler, & Brown, 1992). Being sexually abused as a child (by 15 years of age) apparently leads to a greater likelihood of criminal behavior than do later experiences (Burnam et al., 1988). Likewise, the greater the frequency of childhood sexual victimization among both boys and girls (Dembo et al., 1989, 1992), the more types of sexual abuse endured by girls, and the longer such abuse was endured, the greater the likelihood of subsequent problems (Briere & Zaidi, 1989; Miller, Downs, Gondoli, & Keli, 1987). Other factors that increase the probability of future problems are extended sexual abuse, victimization that involves bizarre acts, multiple perpetrators, and concomitant physical abuse (Briere, 1988; Office of Technology Assessment, 1990). Finally, while more women than men have been sexually assaulted as children, some findings suggest that men may be more likely to develop severe problems as a response to this victimization. Although Burnam et al. (1988) speculate that this may be true because the role of victim is so antithetical to male gender expectations, more research is clearly needed.

Investigators are only beginning to explore why physical abuse and sexual abuse so greatly increase vulnerability to subsequent problems. Briere (1988) believes that victims feel stigmatized by the abuse and that the stigmatization becomes part of their images of themselves. He further suggests that, particularly if a child has experienced high degrees of humiliation, "the child may come to the conclusion that she or he must 'deserve' such treatment, and therefore must be as disgusting and abhorrent as whatever was done to her or him" (p. 332). There is clear evidence that childhood abuse lowers self-esteem and causes self-derogation, and it is thought that these self-image effects help mediate the relationship between the child abuse and subsequent problems. Compared to nonabused children, both abused children *and* children who merely witness instead of experience violence apparently more often cling to adults, complain of loneliness, feel unloved, feel unhappy or sad, and worry a lot (Jaffe, Wolfe, Wilson, & Zak, 1986). Thus family therapists can keep in mind that sad and depressed children may have these "secrets" in their past. Another link between physical/sexual abuse and subsequent substance abuse may be the disturbing thoughts and "flashbacks" of victims (many of whom qualify for a diagnosis of posttraumatic stress disorder), and the wish to avoid these phenomena that victims often report (Rohsenow, Corbett, & Devine, 1988; Wolfe, Gentile, Michienzi, Sas, & Wolfe, 1991). Substance abuse and delinquency may aid victims in "forgetting" their experiences for brief periods of time.

The prevalence of problems in victimized children may also be influenced by other risky parenting practices that appear to coexist with abuse. Abusive parents often spend significantly less time talking to their children, make fewer positive comments, and spend less time teaching the children or joining the children in play. Instead, they spend more time, compared to nonabusive parents, passively looking at or not attending to their children; they also react less often to the children's speech than do nonabusive parents (Kavanagh, Youngblade, Reid, & Fagot, 1988). As a consequence, abused children may be relatively insensitive to social disapproval of conduct problems, because they have not learned to be guided in their actions by responsive parents.

Abusing Substances

The preponderance of evidence indicates that parents' substance abuse produces a manyfold greater risk of problems in their children. Parents' drinking and drug use, including cigarette use, apparently influence the whole range of their children's behaviors. The explanation for this relationship, however, is by no means so clear. As Sher, Walitzer, Wood, and Brent (1991) suggest, researchers are coming to suspect multiple pathways between parental substance abuse and child problems. Some of the relevant correlates of parental substance abuse, in varying combinations for different individuals, are as follows: substances' availability to children, modeling and social learning influences on children, the difficult temperaments of children of substance abusers, and inadequate parenting by substance abusers. Many family therapy clients have these histories—both the parents and the children.

Parents' substance use provides their children with easy access to substances. Except for peers, relatives are young people's most common suppliers of substances, either directly or indirectly (Beier, 1990). Unlocked home liquor storage areas and family medicine cabinets are common sources of young people's substances. The role of learning based on modeling is strongly suggested by repeated findings of similarities between adolescent and adult use patterns (Barnes & Welte, 1990; Brook, Whiteman, Cohen, & Tanaka, 1991). Such modeling of drug use can begin very early, as indicated by evidence that the young sons of male alcoholics tend to be able to differentiate alcoholic from nonalcoholic beverages in photographs and to name the alcoholic beverages, even at 3 years old (Zucker, Kincaid, Fitzgerald, & Bingham, 1994). There is also evidence that children of alcoholics are more likely to think that the purpose of drinking is to get drunk (Newcomb, Huba, & Bentler, 1983) and to have higher expectations that alcohol will enhance their performances (Sher et al., 1991).

In addition, children of substance abusers often appear to display temperamental difficulties from birth, such as heightened arousability, decreased soothability, and negative mood states (Tartar, Alterman, & Edwards, 1985). It may help caretakers of these young people feel more empathy for them to know that they may have been born with these problems. Whether caused by genetic predisposition or congenital problems associated with parental substance use, or both, this difficult temperament—along with the inadequate parenting that can be provided by a substance-abusing parent—has a significant chance of resulting in severe behavior problems (Fitzgerald et al., 1993; Jansen, Fitzgerald, Ham, & Zucker, 1995). Young adult children of alcoholics display "behavioral undercontrol" (impulsivity) that is apparently related to their parents' alcohol problems (Sher et al., 1991).

Research reveals that parental substance abuse is correlated with a significant amount of disruption in child rearing, even in a nonclinical, community sample. Parental substance abuse seems to decrease family cohesion and closeness; to increase family conflict; and to decrease family sociability, expressiveness, pride, and democracy (Senchak, Leonard, Greene, & Carroll, 1995; Tubman, 1991). Parents who abuse substances have been found to have unrealistically high expectations of their children and to think that they should be competent at a number of tasks much earlier than other parents think this (Kumpfer & DeMarsh, 1986). These parents are apparently also inconsistent in protective parenting practices, such as nurturing, involvement in their children's lives, attention to their children's feelings, positive guidance, and supervision (Chassin, Pillow, Curran, Molina, & Barrera, 1993; Dishion et al., 1988; Kumpfer & DeMarsh, 1986; Jones & Houts, 1992). As an apparent consequence, children of substance abusers show less social attachment and involvement, and have difficulties getting along with other children (Johnson & Pandina, 1991). Because of parents' difficulties in family management and supervision, children of substance abusers are often absent or late to school, are often poorly fed and clothed, and receive little help with their schoolwork (Kumpfer & DeMarsh, 1986). They also experience more stressful life events, such as changing residences (Valliant & Milofsky, 1982); parental unemployment, divorce, illness, and death (Tubman, 1991); and poverty (El-Guebaly & Offord, 1977).

There seems to be a linear relationship between the length of time parents are involved with substances and the developmental and social problems of their young children (Johnson, Glassman, Fiks, & Rosen, 1990). Substance abuse in one spouse may impair the parenting behavior of the other; for instance, spouses of alcohol abusers are often depressed, isolated from other adults, and so involved with their substance-abusing partners that children feel neglected (Benson & Heller, 1987). Marital satisfaction can be low (Tubman, 1991), and the marital relationship can include significant verbal and physical aggression (Straus & Sweet, 1992).

Finally, experiments have shown that even in parents without substance use problems, the use of substances can disrupt ongoing parenting behavior. There is evidence that *any* parent who consumes three or four drinks is less attentive to and notices less of a child's behavior; is less task-oriented; and is less consistent with a child than usual, simultaneously increasing both commands and indulgences (Lang, 1992).

In sum, parenting that involves neglect, physical abuse, sexual victimization, or substance abuse increases the risk of problems in offspring. These risk factors in children's lives create loneliness, social rejection, and painful memories, while simultaneously depriving them of protective factors—reinforcing close relationships, parental monitoring, and training in effective functioning both in the home and in the larger world.

EFFECTIVENESS OF PROACTIVE FAMILY INTERVENTIONS

In this section, we describe empirically investigated, proactive family interventions. We proceed from interventions beginning at birth or early childhood to those administered during middle childhood and adolescence. Within each group, the more universally applicable interventions are discussed first, followed by the more selective or indicated interventions.

Empirically Supported Family Interventions for Early Childhood Problems

Longitudinal data suggest that child- and caregiver-focused interventions that are targeted, intensive, long-term, and comprehensive can increase protective factors and improve positive outcomes for children. Studies of such interventions have included eastern U.S. Blacks, Whites, and Hispanics; midwestern U.S. Blacks and Whites; and California Blacks, Whites, and Hispanics. In successful interventions, professionals do not assume parents' responsibilities, but support their efforts at protective parenting, increasing their skill and confidence. Some of the elements of successful multicomponent early interventions are (1) providing parents with child care support; (2) assessing with parents their children's progress over time, and discussing normative developmental expectations regularly at a time and place convenient for parents (often the home); and (3) providing the parents with other adults to talk to about parenting—adults who empathize with and normalize feelings of incompetence, who know resources and coping methods, and who collaborate with the parents in gaining access to community services for their children.

The Yale Child Welfare Research Program, the Perry Preschool Project, and Project 12-Ways are notable examples of successful early intervention programs for at-risk children. "Successful," in this context, means that programs have measurably improved child outcomes, at a total cost savings to taxpayers. The Yale Child Welfare Research Program has yielded evidence that 30 months of home-based intervention beginning when impoverished mothers were pregnant with their first child significantly increased protective parental warmth, parental monitoring of schoolwork, and parental help seeking and collaboration with children's teachers *for at least 10 years*, compared to a matched nonintervention group (Seitz, 1990; Seitz, Rosenbaum, & Apfel, 1985). Poor Black, White, and Hispanic women were recruited into the intervention in a northeastern hospital clinic and received regular pediatric care, home visitors, optional day care, and regular developmental examinations for their children. The resulting improvements both in parenting practices and in the children's language development and school adjustment supported the Yale program's assumptions that "by working with each family for a sufficient length of time, the particular problems most in need of attention could be determined and dealt with—and, in turn, if parents' own lives could be improved, their children would also benefit" (Seitz, 1990, p. 84). Not only did parents and children benefit, but the taxpayers did so as well. By the 10-year follow-up, special school services such as remedial education and court hearings had cost $1,120 a year less for each intervention child than for each nonintervention child.

Another controlled, longitudinal study provided low-income midwestern Black parents with 1–2 years of high-quality early education for their 3- and 4-year-olds, arranged frequent 30 minute home visits from the children's teachers for discussion of the children's education, and set up parent groups that met monthly to exchange views and support for child rearing. This intervention, the Perry Preschool Project of the High/Scope Educational Research Foundation, lowered several substance abuse risk factors in the youth over a 16-year period; it also resulted in improved high school graduation and employment rates, as well as reduced arrests (Berrueta-Clement, Schweinhart, Barnett, & Weikart, 1987). Analyses showed that in court costs alone, the early intervention saved taxpayers $2,400 per child (Barnett & Escobar, 1990). Although this intervention research did not measure parenting, it is hypothesized that the Perry Preschool Project group outperformed the control group because while the children were in preschool, their parents became comfortable collaborating with their children's teachers. As a result, they learned to keep track of their children's academic progress and to contact teachers subsequently throughout the children's schooling (Seitz, 1990). These changes in behavior can, of course, be seen as the development of monitoring and advocacy, which are two of the protective parenting skills described above.

A third field trial has indicated that even parental neglect and child abuse can be altered through intervention. In a multifaceted, home-based intervention called Project 12-Ways, predominantly White midwestern parents were referred to the project by the state child protective agency due to indications of child abuse or neglect. Their 3- to 9-year-old children were at risk of being removed from the home (which would have involved the difficulties and costs of foster care, divided families, etc.). After in-home assessment and consultation with each family, a family counselor provided the following components for 1 year, as needed: parent–child interaction training; social support; health and nutrition maintenance; training in home safety, problem solving, stress reduction, and financial management; job search counseling; alcoholism treatment referral; and assertiveness training (Lutzker, Campbell, Newman, & Harrold, 1989). Repeated comparisons of these parents' recidivism rates with those of "service-as-usual" parents suggested that Project 12-Ways parents were significantly less likely to injure or neglect their children (Lutzker & Rice, 1987). Although one study (Wesch & Lutzker, 1991) indicated that booster sessions might be needed to maintain these rates, the finding that Project 12-Ways could lower a state's monthly expense for high-risk children from $315 to $265 (California State Council on Developmental Disabilities, 1989) indicated that this intervention would be well worth continued investigation.

Empirically Supported Family Interventions for Middle Childhood Problems

Upon entering school, children may encounter academic, social, and behavioral difficulties that can lead to negative life trajectories (Dishion et al., 1988). Evidence shows that altering parenting practices can reduce these problems. Some programs are available to all parents of school-age children, while other programs target parents with serious identified parenting problems, such as substance abuse. Empirically supported home-based and community-based interventions often target multiple influences in the children's lives simultaneously and over a long period of time. They support and improve parenting through external interventions, such as parent meetings, home visitors, and telephone calls; train teachers to support parent efforts; and teach children more adaptive social and communication skills. Program workers gain access to parents by going to places that they naturally frequent. For parents of children in this age group, the critical protective parenting skills seem to be positive communication, behavior management, and involvement in children's lives outside the home.

The Seattle Social Skills Development Project, a sophisticated parenting intervention aimed at all parents of elementary school children, was tested for 4 years in eight Seattle public schools (Hawkins, Catalano, Morrison et al., 1992; Hawkins, Von Cleve, & Catalano, 1991). Parents received two components, the first consisting of a seven-session group parent training curriculum called "Catch 'Em Being Good," which was offered when their children entered first grade and again when they entered second grade. In the spring of each of these school years, parents were offered a second component, a four-session group parent training curriculum entitled "How to Help Your Child Succeed in School." In the first grade, children were taught interpersonal cognitive problem-solving skills (Shure & Spivack, 1988). Teachers were trained in positive methods to promote appropriate behavior and learning, and to make learning enjoyable.

Through multiple, varied, repeated community-based recruiting methods (see Hawkins, Catalano, & Associates, 1992), parents of approximately 47% of the Seattle students volunteered to attend at least one class. Parents tended to return after their initial session; mean attendance at "Catch 'Em Being Good" was for 78% of the sessions and at "How to Help Your Child Succeed in School" was for 90% of the sessions. Forty percent of the attendees were single parents, 46% were from low-income families, and 52% were members of ethnic minority groups.

By the fall of fifth grade, this coordinated intervention had resulted in improved parental behavior management practices and family communication, greater family closeness, and more parental involvement with the school for fifth-grade parents in schools receiving the intervention, whether or not they attended parent training. This increased protective parenting in turn lowered their children's problems. Their children reported increased pleasure in and commitment to school, decreased initiation of delinquency, and less initiation of substance use (Hawkins, Catalano, Morrison et al., 1992).

The Montreal Longitudinal–Experimental Study, which also offered coordinated parenting and child social skills training in first and second grades, yielded even longer-term evidence that this approach could reduce delinquency, including substance use (Tremblay, Pagani-Kurtz, Mosse, Vitaro, & Pihl, 1995). French-speaking, lower-socioeconomic-status boys selected because of disruptive behavior in kindergarten received school-based social skills training during first and second grades, while their parents were offered 2 years of individualized, home-based parent training based on the Oregon Social Learning Center model (Patterson et al., 1975). Although Tremblay et al. (1995) did not specify the effects of training on parenting behavior, they found that from 1 through 6 years after this multicomponent intervention ended (when the boys were from 10 through 15 years old), the boys in the experimental group reported significantly fewer delinquent acts, including substance use, than did the boys who were randomly assigned to a no-intervention group. Tremblay et al. (1995) suggested that booster sessions might further enhance intervention effects, for although gains in other behaviors were maintained, initial positive effects on academic performance faded after 3 years.

Findings on the Strengthening Families Program (Kumpfer, 1990) suggested that even hard-to-reach parents who displayed few initial protective practices could learn better parenting through persistent, respectful coaching. Designed to benefit selected 6- to 12-year-old children of substance abusers and other at-risk children, the program provided 14 group sessions that involved parenting training, youth skills training, and family skills training. Transportation and meals were provided to encourage training attendance. Taken together, the three coordinated interventions apparently improved parents' behavior management skills and family relationships, which in turn decreased alcohol and drug use in older children.

Empirically Supported Family Interventions for Adolescent Problems

The adolescent years bring new developmental tasks. Because adolescents spend less time under their parents' supervision, protective parenting involves less direct behavior management at home and more indirect influence through involvement, advocacy, and help seeking outside of the home. As is true at previous developmental stages, the most effective parenting interventions for parents of adolescents (those that have been documented to reduce school and behavior problems) seem to be multisystemic—aimed at influencing more than one aspect of adolescents' social setting. New parenting behaviors are reinforced and supported by program personnel, who take a collaborative stance that respects both what parents are already doing well and their autonomy as adults.

Rodick and Henggeler (1980) found clear evidence that short-term weekly outreach (10 weeks) to parents of high-risk early adolescents both increased protective parenting practices and reduced poor academic achievement. Mature university students contacted parents of the lowest-achieving seventh-graders in a midwestern inner-city school serving low-income Black youth, and helped the parents plan to devote 1 hour an evening to reading or doing homework with their children. The university students then monitored and facilitated parental involvement through weekly telephone calls and biweekly home visits. Not only was the academic achievement of the adolescents improved at the end of the 10-week intervention, but the improvement continued for a year afterward. Thus family practitioners can have a long-term positive impact if all they manage to do is motivate parents to do homework with their children.

Dishion and Andrews's (1995) Adolescent Transition Program has provided further evidence that strategies based entirely on outreach and behavioral support for parents can produce long-term gains in protective parenting of adolescents. White, middle-class parents of high-risk youth in the northwestern United States were recruited through media advertisements, school flyers, and community agencies for 12 weekly parenting sessions, both group and individualized. Parents were taught to communicate clear, consistent "house rules" and appropriate consequences for infractions. Videotapes of behavior at home showed that parents reduced their negative communications with their children by the end of the intervention, as compared with parents in other interventions or a no-intervention condition. Their adolescents responded by behaving better at home and in school (although school effects faded in 1 year), and by using less tobacco than other high risk youth.

Krinsley (1991) found evidence that providing 3–4 months of Bry's home-based Targeted Family Intervention plus booster sessions (Bry & Krinsley, 1992), in combination with Bry's (1982) previously tested school-based Early Secondary Intervention Program, could significantly reduce school failure and initiation of substance use for at least 2 years among high-risk seventh- and eighth-graders. School personnel in an ethnically mixed, working-class northeastern U.S. town identified youth who exhibited poor academic performance and behavior problems, and asked parents' permission to refer the youth to a program for "students who could do better in school." The youth and the families, in separate sessions, were given weekly feedback by behavioral family therapists about the students' progress in school. The youth and families also discussed together with the family counselors how parents could influence the youth's behavior more positively. Krinsley's study has been replicated successfully in a predominantly Black, low-income northeastern U.S. community by Alexander (1997).

Borduin et al. (1995) measured which family variables changed as their multisystemic family therapy reduced adolescent problems in very high-risk, lower-income, midwestern Black and White juvenile offenders. The researchers found evidence that a mean of 24 hours of their home-based, child-centered, family-focused, comprehensive, and flexible intervention increased family cohesion and adaptability, increased parents' support for their adolescents and for each other, decreased conflict and hostility, and decreased parental psychiatric symptoms (e.g., depression). The measured long-term effect on the juvenile offenders was a dramatic reduction in recidivism (26% vs. the usual 71%) for at least 4 years after treatment. Schmidt, Liddle, and Dakof (1996) also measured improvements in parenting while families were in their multidimensional family therapy for adolescent drug use and behavior problems (Liddle, Dakof, & Diamond, 1991). Taken together, these studies show that reaching out to families proactively can reduce both risky parenting practices and subsequent behavior problems among high-risk adolescents.

Not only are multisystems family approaches effective, but they also save money. Despite its intensity, multisystemic family therapy is relatively inexpensive. In 1992, Henggeler, Melton, and Smith reported that multisystemic family therapy reduced arrests and incarceration days in a randomly assigned group of juvenile offenders in Simpsonville, North Carolina, and that it cost just $2,800 per adolescent. In contrast, the average cost of institutional placement at that time in North Carolina was $16,300. In a less controlled study, Henggeler, Melton, Brondino, Schere, and Hanley (1997) calculated that over a 2-year period, multisystemic family therapy, in comparison with usual services, reduced incarceration by 74.4 days per client. At $100 a day for institutionalization, $7,440 per client was saved by providing this form of therapy.

DISCUSSION

Research in the past decade has yielded consistent evidence that parenting practices can either increase risk for child problems or serve as protective factors against them, across cultural and ethnic groups and across developmental stages. Protective factors—such as parental warmth, monitoring, positive behavioral management, involvement in children's activities outside the home, and social support seeking—probably work by limiting children's access to deviant friends and activities, promoting involvement in constructive activities, and providing sanctions against delinquent behavior. On the other hand, it seems clear that risk factors—such as parental neglect, perpetration of sexual and physical abuse, or parental substance abuse—can increase children's access to substances, increase their exposure to traumatic experiences from which they wish to escape, and diminish parents' ability to influence their children against delinquency. Family practitioners will want to encourage families to increase protective factors and eliminate risk factors.

Furthermore, taken together, studies by a variety of researchers suggest that parenting behavior can be altered effectively by proactive family interventions. Furthermore, it is clear that effective programs are well received by participants. Effective family interventions are multifaceted and usually last a long time—from 3 months to 2 years of a child's life. They support the positive goals that parents have for their children. They build on whatever protective practices are present, by acknowledging and praising the skills parents already exhibit. Parents do not have to perceive themselves as failures or as needing help to receive program benefits. Parents generally participate because they want their children to have a specific opportunity, such as day care or help in school. Programs typically focus on specific child behaviors (e.g., schoolwork) that parents can observe and that concern parents.

Most parents would like to be more effective in guiding their children toward constructive ways of life. Parents who feel powerless, stressed, and incompetent are more likely to engage in risky parenting practices such as coercive behavior management. Thus, by and large, family practitioners can promote protective parenting by increasing parents' sense of control, their sense that their problems are manageable, and their personal competence. They do this by providing parents with social and practical resources, such as other adults with whom they can share the responsibilities of raising their children (as partners or collaborators) and the necessary knowledge and support to seek out community services and institutions that support healthy child rearing. Although several of these interventions benefit the parents directly, parents' basic motivation to participate seems to be based on their hopes for their children, not for themselves.

There now exists ample research information upon which to base proactive home-based family, school, and community interventions. The time when practitioners had to work in the dark is past. Our review of the research shows that effective family interventions typically seem to have two or more of the following components:

- Expert social support (trained family therapists and group leaders).

- Personalized partners in meeting parents' individual goals for their children and families (e.g., individualized, multisystemic, family-based counseling).
- Multiple sessions of a manualized parent skills curriculum, with videotapes and handouts covering specific problems (e.g., how to help with homework, how to handle a child's fears).
- Assessment and monitoring of children's development.
- Empowerment and training in advocacy (e.g., information about how to talk to special education personnel about children's learning problems).
- Information that parents value (e.g., information about summer youth job opportunities, normative developmental expectations, or ways to protect children from crime, school failure, or substance abuse).
- Simultaneous group or individual behavioral counseling for children (e.g., academic skills, mediation skills to avoid gang fighting, behavioral counseling).

CHAPTER 11

Supervision and Training

Just as our therapeutic methods draw heavily on the empowerment of clients, our supervisory philosophy is based on the empowerment of family therapists and supervisors. In order for family therapists to be able to see strengths in the families they treat, supervisors must model that approach. For family workers overburdened with the demands of large caseloads, the pressures of managed care, and the challenge of families who present with many life stressors (Berg, 1994; Boyd-Franklin, 1989; Kagan & Schlossberg, 1989), a supervisory process that focuses on the positive can serve as a life preserver.

Just as parents who feel accused, blamed, and judged by family workers tend to blame and scapegoat their children and adolescents, therapists who feel blamed and unsupported by their supervisors tend to be harsh in judging or diagnosing the clients and families they treat. In this respect, our model of supportive supervision is not only an investment in the personal and professional development of family therapists, but it also has a direct link to clinical outcome (Boyd-Franklin, 1989). This chapter presents an in-depth exploration of supervisory and training techniques that will enable workers to do their jobs (i.e., help the families they treat to achieve goals) without suffering the burnout that all too often accompanies the treatment of families burdened with severe circumstances.

THE NEED FOR AN ORIENTATION PROCESS

As stated previously, agencies are under pressure to handle caseloads and often have difficulty finding the time for an orientation process for new staff members. This should include orientation to agency policies, but it should also be used to assess the new worker's strengths and weaknesses and to provide additional training when necessary. It is also helpful if a manual can be developed that provides a careful overview of information new workers will need. Guidelines for safety in home-based work should definitely be included. (See Chapter 3).

With the rapid turnover of therapists in some agencies, new family workers may be expected to function without the benefit of this thorough orientation. In the best-case scenario, clinicians seek out more senior workers in their agency. In the worst-case scenario, because of caseload demands, they are forced to begin immediately with a large number of families and little preparation.

As indicated earlier, in addition to the need for an actual orientation, clinicians also a need supervisors who take a very "hands-on," "front-line" approach to supervision, and who are available and can be reached when crises develop.

FRONT-LINE SUPERVISION

The multisystems model, including home-based family, school, and community interventions, requires a very active treatment approach in which outreach plays a vital part. This can occur on many levels. As discussed in Chapters 2 and 8, because of the "resistance," hesitation, and suspicion of many communities toward mental health treatment, credibility must be established on a community level, as well as on a case-by-case level. Therefore, it is very important for agency directors and clinical supervisors to have a front-line presence in the community or communities they serve. As workers change over time, supervisors and administrators can then become a bridge and "introduce" new workers into a community. Often it is helpful for supervisors to take a front-line role by going out on early home visits with new staff members. This first level of front-line supervision is often omitted by many agencies; others engage in community outreach only in the initial stages of the establishment of a new service, but fail to follow through by maintaining *ongoing* contact with the community.

One method of front-line supervision and administration that addresses the need for ongoing contact is "networking," whereby someone in a position of authority in an agency is well connected to key leaders and resources within the community. This serves many purposes. First, it can help to establish the positive "word of mouth" crucial to an agency's credibility. Second, designating one person to maintain ongoing contacts in the community will ensure that the agency is acting with up-to-date information, since it is not possible for each individual family worker to have key contacts in each multisystems agency, let alone to be cognizant of each agency's personnel changes. As shown in Chapter 8, knowledge of a key participant in the community can be invaluable to a family worker who must negotiate one of these complex systems in partnership with a client or family.

Another component of front-line supervision is that supervisors and agency administrators know the families and communities they serve. We have found it very useful as supervisors to make occasional home visits with our supervisees, to initiate and attend meetings with community agencies, and to work in partnership with other community programs on shared grant proposals or collaborative community initiatives.

For clinicians to feel competent and supported in the "hands-on" work this treatment approach requires, it is essential that supervisors and agency administrators model this philosophy. For example, when a support group is being organized in a local community, supervisors can colead the first few group sessions; this will help them to understand the issues that supervisees encounter, and to join with the community and establish a visible presence there.

For new staff members and students, it is also often helpful for a supervisor or a senior, more experienced family worker to accompany them on their first few home visits and/or multisystems meetings, in order to support and observe. Later, the supervisor or senior worker can give direct, nonjudgmental, and supportive supervisory input about the new worker's home-based family intervention skills.

Another opportunity to engage in hands-on supervision occurs when a family is in crisis. We often utilize these occasions to do a consultation session with a supervisee about a client or family, especially since a family crisis presents an opportunity for change. A supervisor or consulting clinician should be careful not to undermine the credibility or power of the family worker or of the parental figures in the family. The manner in which this is broached to the family or client should stress the collaborative efforts of all parties to find a solution. It might be expressed in this way: "With your permission, I would like to invite Dr. _____, my supervisor, to come out and meet with us for our next home-based session. We can brainstorm together about how to solve this problem."

It is also often helpful to invite a family to come in for a "live interview" at the agency or clinic, in which the supervisor or consultant can meet with the family worker and the family to explore solutions to a particular issue. Once again, it is essential that this be proposed within a collegial, collaborating framework. It is particularly important for new staff members or student trainees not to undermine their credibility with their clients by presenting themselves as needing the intercession of supervisors and consultants, or by communicating that they occupy a low position in the agency hierarchy. (Observing this type of interview can also be very instructive for students and trainees, so holding it in a room with a one-way mirror, or videotaping with the family's consent, might be pursued.)

Front-line supervision also requires enhanced availability on the part of supervisors, as well as a process for emergency consultations. Many of the clients discussed in this book have very difficult life circumstances, and crises do not occur on a convenient 9-to-5 schedule. It is important that a mechanism be developed for handling such occurrences on evenings and weekends. Some programs contract with a local emergency room or crisis intervention unit. Others establish a system in which different staff members or supervisors are "on call" on a rotating basis. It is important that supervisors and key administrators also be available for consultation in these circumstances.

It is crucial, however, to be mindful that staff members also need protection within this model of front-line supervision. Endless "on-call" days can lead to burnout and undermine the effectiveness of both staff and supervisors. As previously explained in Chapter 8, some agencies have established "comp time," so that workers who involve themselves in a family's crisis regardless of their work schedule may be reimbursed by coming in later or leaving earlier when the crisis abates. In order for a "comp time" program to be successful, a system of record keeping must be developed and maintained.

THE MANAGEMENT OF CRISES

Throughout this book, we have shown how crises can often serve a purpose for clients and families. It is also important to understand the function that repetitive crises often serve for family workers. Some family workers, particularly early in their careers, find that solving crises puts them in a position of power vis-à-vis their clients. They begin to feel competent in the work and feel validated for offering a much-needed service. Often younger workers feel the need to be seen as change agents by family members, and are very empowered by this process. This can also occur with experienced family workers. Well-meaning clinicians can inadvertently fall into the trap of always responding in "crisis mode," as indicated in Chapter 4.

An important supervisory issue in many of these cases is the process of helping family workers to explore their own role in repetitive crises. The need to feel empowered by the "solving" of a family crisis may occur at the expense of the empowerment of the client or family (Kagan & Schlossberg, 1989). It is also crucial for staff members to be aware of what constitutes an actual crisis. An anxious student, trainee, or worker may respond to a family's definition of a "crisis" without determining whether this is a true emergency.

OTHER SUPERVISORY DILEMMAS

Helping Workers to Confront Clients When Necessary

Another supervisory dilemma that can occur often with new or inexperienced family workers is their need to be loved and appreciated by their clients. In the initial stages of treatment, this need may result in positive consequences: It can facilitate joining and lead to the development of a good initial therapeutic alliance, in which clients show up regularly for sessions. Often, however, an "excellent" relationship comes at a price: Despite the family's regular attendance at meetings with a worker, no change is occurring, or there is a major therapeutic impasse around a treatment issue. The challenge for the supervisee and supervisor is to identify the impasse and explore the issues getting in the way for both the family and the clinician in the process of producing change.

Even an experienced clinician often finds himself or herself in a dilemma when the therapist has worked hard to establish a therapeutic bond with a client and family, but begins to suspect that a family member "in recovery" may be experiencing a relapse in drug or alcohol addiction. There is often a fear that a confrontation will disrupt this therapeutic alliance. Once again, timing, sensitivity, and the framing of such an intervention are crucial in both the clinical and the supervisory process.

Case Example

Barbara McMann (age 40) and her family were referred for treatment by child protective services because workers at that agency were concerned that Barbara's substance abuse might be interfering with her parenting and leading to neglect of her children. This Irish American family included Mark (age 15), Beverly (age 10), and Carl (age 5). The family was supported by public assistance and was living in a trailer park. The child protective service workers informed Barbara that if she was not able to overcome her addiction to cocaine and maintain her recovery, her children would be removed from her home.

The family worker joined with Barbara and learned of her strong desire to keep her family together. After 2 months of sessions, the family worker was able to convince her to go into a drug detox program, and subsequently to attend an inpatient rehab program for 28 days. The family worker also helped Barbara in a session to negotiate with her mother to keep her children for the length of these programs. Before her entry into the detox program, a family session was held in which Barbara explained to her children what she would be doing, and told them that they would be in their grandmother's care while she was on the inpatient detox and rehab units. With the family worker's help, she frankly answered their questions about her addiction.

After her discharge, Barbara appeared to be a new person. She took her recovery very seriously and attended an outpatient rehab program and a number of Twelve-Step (Narcotics Anonymous) meetings per week. She also became more actively involved in parenting her children and in the home-based family therapy sessions.

Barbara had been in recovery for about 5 months when a crisis occurred: Her mother, who had been a major support to her, died suddenly of a heart attack. The signs of her relapse were subtle at first. Barbara began canceling family sessions. The family worker, who had grown very close to Barbara and her children, felt very sorry about Barbara's loss. She admired her recovery struggle and missed the signs of Barbara's relapse that her mother's death precipitated.

In addition to Barbara's canceling family sessions, she stopped attending her recovery groups. After 3 weeks of Barbara's cancelled sessions, the family worker met with her supervisor, who worked with the therapist to recognize the signs of her relapse. The family worker was able to talk honestly about her fears of addressing this issue with Barbara; she was apprehensive that she might endanger the therapeutic alliance with her. The supervisor helped the family worker to role-play some ways to confront Barbara in a positive but direct way about her return to substance use. The emphasis was placed on Barbara's wish as a mother for a drug-free, positive life for her children. They also discussed the importance of the family worker's emphasizing her caring for Barbara and her children.

With this direct supervisory help, the family worker was able to confront Barbara positively, get past her denials of her current substance use, and convince her to enter a drug detox and rehab center that would provide housing and support groups for her and her children. This was very important to Barbara, as she did not want to lose custody of her children while she sought help.

Cultural and Racial Issues in Supervision

With the ever-increasing diversity in the United States, therapists are constantly faced with new clients from cultures different from their own (Gibbs & Huang, 1998). This will lead to an increased likelihood of cross-cultural and/or cross-racial treatment (Comas-Díaz & Griffiths,

1988; McGoldrick et al., 1996). As more ethnic minority therapists and supervisors enter the field, there is also an increased likelihood of cross-cultural or cross-racial supervision (Helms & Cook, 1999).

In recent years, the process of cross-cultural and cross-racial treatment has been studied (Carter, 1990; Carter & Helms, 1992). Although still in its early stages, research in this area has grown in recent years (Helms & Cook, 1999; Sue, Arredondo, & McDavis, 1992; Sue & Sue, 1990; Sue & Zane, 1987, Sue, Zane, & Young, 1994). The issues related to cross-cultural supervision, however, are still in their infancy (Boyd-Franklin, 1989; Hardy, 1989). Many training programs in family therapy, social work, psychology, and psychiatry have functioned for years with what Hardy (1989) describes as the "theoretical myth of sameness . . . or the belief that all families [or clients] are virtually the same" (p. 18). Hardy has successfully challenged these beliefs—a position wholeheartedly endorsed by Helms and Cook (1999), who state:

> The cultural orientation or predisposition of each of the participants in the [therapy] process—supervisor, supervisee, and client(s)—may also be invisible, but is a meaningful dynamic in supervision. . . . We think Hardy's points about therapy supervision pertain to the therapy process more globally as well as to the supervisor–supervisee relationship regardless of whether the therapist–client relationship involves families, other kinds of groups, or individual clients. (p. 291)

A number of supervisors have given guidelines for cross-cultural and cross-racial supervision (Boyd-Franklin, 1989; Helms & Cook, 1999; Hunt, 1987). Hunt (1987) was one of the first authors to document supervisory issues for Black and White therapists working with black clients. Boyd-Franklin (1989) has presented a number of guidelines for supervisors of Black and White therapists working with Black families. The chapters "Therapist's Use of Self and Value Conflicts with Black Families" (Chapter 6) and "Implications for Training and Supervision" (Chapter 14) both explore these issues for supervisors and therapists of different ethnic and racial backgrounds. Supervisors must feel comfortable themselves in raising these issues with supervisees, if the supervisees are to feel comfortable in exploring these issues with their clients and families.

Supervision as a Process of Negotiation

When a supervisor is introduced to a new staff member or family therapist, it often takes time to establish a positive working relationship and to establish an open, honest context in which the family therapist's skills can be evaluated. This is complicated when, as in many clinics and agencies, the supervisor is responsible for evaluations of the supervisee's progress.

Another potential pitfall is a supervisor's inadvertent overestimation or underestimation of a supervisee's experience and competence. A common example of underestimation occurs when clinicians who have had several years of experience in office-based family therapy are doing home-based family treatment for the first time. They will resent being "supervised" as beginners. In many forms of clinical work, supervision is viewed as a hierarchical, power-based relationship with the supervisee in the inferior position. Particularly in the home-based or outreach modality, such structure is contrary to effective treatment progress and to the development of counselors' competence. Experienced office-based therapists who are involved in home-based therapy for the first time will welcome ongoing consultation to assist them in the transition to home-based interventions if it is respectful of their past experience.

It is helpful to approach supervision as a process of negotiation—to frame it as consultation, which implies a partnership and not a hierarchy. Family workers should be encouraged in their first supervisory meetings to talk about their past experiences in the field. They should also be encouraged to discuss what they perceive to be their strengths and the areas where they feel competent. They can then be encouraged to identify areas in which they need help to grow or learn more. During the subsequent evaluation process, supervisors and supervisees can explore and discuss the progress achieved in meeting these goals.

It is also beneficial for supervisors to let clinicians know that their supervisory style is open to input and negotiation. For example, because we currently supervise graduate students who are relatively inexperienced, we have found it useful to be directive in the early stages of supervision. Although this is a very useful strategy with workers who are new to both family therapy and home-based approaches, it can be perceived as condescending or infantilizing by clinicians who have had more treatment experience. Therefore, we have found it helpful to acknowledge our supervisory style in the initial sessions and to let our supervisees know that we see supervision as an ongoing negotiation process geared to facilitate their learning. As they become more confident, supervisees can then take more risks and begin to negotiate the type of supervision that is most helpful and empowering for them at different stages of their own development. This is particularly important for staff members or trainees who have had the same supervisors for many years. Often the shifts in feelings of competence are subtle, and it is helpful for supervisors to discuss this openly with their supervisees. Also, it is helpful for supervisees to experience a number of different supervisors. This can enrich the experience for them.

Mechanisms for Building Skills, Providing Support, and Developing Teamwork

One of the many parallels between supervision and clinical work, as emphasized throughout this book, is that often "helping" is not "empowering." Supervisors should be vigilant about empowering clinicians to take more and more responsibility for developing their own treatment plans and strategies. Four mechanisms, discussed below, are particularly helpful for empowering clinicians through skill building, support provision, and the development of teamwork: (1) hiring an outside consultant; (2) clinical case conferences; (3) multidisciplinary teams; and (4) peer supervision.

The Use of an Outside Consultant

The practice of home-based, school, and community interventions is clearly demanding. Many agencies and programs have handled this dilemma by hiring an outside consultant, as needed, to address specific issues. Outside consultants may be utilized in helping to address organizational issues or staff burnout; to train staff members and supervisors in a specific content area that is new to them; to explore an area of cultural competency with a particular ethnic or racial group; or to offer assistance with cases demanding specific expertise (such as those involving alcoholism and drug abuse, chronic abuse or neglect, child custody, violence, juvenile delinquency, etc.).

Although both of us have had extensive experience in serving as consultants to other programs and agencies and in utilizing consultants in our own clinical and research efforts, we have found it very useful to invite a colleague from outside our project to join us, our staff, and our students to explore a particular issue. We are very grateful to our colleagues who have been willing to consult with us on such issues as community entry, interface with other multisystemic agencies, and partnership with other programs.

Case Conferences

Some agencies have adopted regular case conferences (or, in some instances, "difficult case conferences") in which all staff members, supervisors and administrators work together, sometimes with the help of an outside consultant, to brainstorm the treatment of difficult cases.

These sessions can also serve to establish an atmosphere of ongoing learning and professional development; such a climate can be refreshing and refueling and can serve as an antidote to burnout for all staff, supervisors, administrators, and trainees.

It is helpful to agree on a format for presenting cases at these conferences. Typically, cases are written up or presented orally, or some combination of these is used. In addition, visual aids can be offered: a family tree or genogram (McGoldrick & Gerson, 1985) can be drawn to illustrate multigenerational family patterns; an eco-map (Hartman & Laird, 1983) can be included to show the involvement of the client or family with different multisystems agencies.

Case conference presentations often include the following key areas:

• Presenting problems
• Description of client and family history
• Case diagnoses
• Formulation
• Treatment plan
• Treatment summary
• Questions for discussion

In addition to the knowledge gained in such sessions, important implicit messages are conveyed: We are all in this work together; no one person has all the answers; all of us can learn from each other; asking for help is a positive thing; ongoing learning and training are important for all of us, no matter what our level of experience; and training is an antidote to burnout (Boyd-Franklin, 1989).

Multidisciplinary Teams

One of the advantages of working in the fields of mental health, home-based family intervention, medical and health services, social service, and education is that they often bring together individuals from very diverse professional backgrounds and experiences (teachers, school administrators, psychologists, psychiatrists, other physicians, nurses, social workers, child welfare workers, outreach workers, police, probation officers, judges, etc.). These individuals often approach a problem from very different perspectives. Although such diversity can often lead to misunderstandings and difficulties in communication, it can also be a very enriching experience.

Because front-line family workers are often out in the field, they may feel isolated and miss the opportunity to connect regularly with colleagues. Unlike agencies or programs in which clinicians work in the same office and the clientele comes in for treatment, home- or community-based workers can sometimes feel disconnected from the work of others and need a sense of a "home base" of their own. Staff meetings and multidisciplinary team meetings can serve the purpose of countering isolation and can reinforce the sense of connectedness to the project or program. Multidisciplinary team meetings offer different professional perspectives on a problem. If these meetings are held regularly (possibly in combination with regular case conferences), they can contribute greatly to the process of team building.

These team meetings are also an excellent time to share resources, including contacts with individuals in other agencies. Staff members can interact with colleagues trained in different family therapy models, or more individually focused behavioral, cognitive-behavioral, or psychodynamic approaches. Team meetings also present an excellent opportunity to identify the "agency experts" on different multisystems institutions. For example, a social worker with considerable child welfare experience may be able to help staff members interact more effectively with child protective services. A psychiatrist with years of hospital-based experience may be able to help nonpsychiatric mental health workers to interact and understand the medical terminology of other physicians. If this sort of interaction takes place within a collaborative, supportive framework, multidisciplinary team meetings can be enriching for all involved.

For administrators, these meetings can serve both a team-building and an organizational purpose. They provide an opportunity to discuss intake cases with staff members and to discuss treatment plans. They serve the purpose of helping to orient new staff members and trainees to the "culture of the program." Finally, they provide an opportunity to strategize about issues affecting the entire agency, such as funding, managed care, census of clients, and new programs and directions for the agency.

Peer Supervision

In the current atmosphere of budget cuts and managed care demands, "supervision" can constitute little more than administrative monitoring of required paperwork at its worst, and case management at its best. Limitations on the process of supervision decrease the clinical effectiveness of the family work and may increase the likelihood of staff burnout. In home-based family treatment, and in all multisystems work, even experienced workers need ongoing clinical case supervision and consultation.

Family workers, particularly at social service agencies, may experience "supervision" as administrative monitoring, rather than a process of receiving regular clinical or case supervision. Other agencies may provide excellent case supervision for students, interns, and trainees, but may abruptly discontinue the supervision once the family workers have completed training.

Given the realities of today's front-line environment, however, family workers should be prepared for the possibility that their agency may not provide adequate supervision. One way to counter this deficit is for family workers to form peer supervision groups with other workers from their own agency, or possibly from other agencies. This can be planned around lunchtime: Everyone can bring a brown-bag lunch and spend an hour once a week discussing cases. The case conference format discussed above can also be utilized, or a more informal structure can be tried. It is essential, however, that meetings be regularly scheduled. It is helpful for meetings to be arranged for an entire year in advance, so that participants reserve those dates on their calendars. If lunchtime meetings don't work out because of competing schedules, some workers have found it beneficial to arrange early morning or after-work meetings once per week. Even if they are scheduled for once or twice per month, sessions can be extremely helpful if they meet the two necessary conditions of regularity and predictability.

Family workers often underestimate the value of peer supervision: One does not need an "expert" in order to learn; regular case discussions sharpen the clinical skills of all workers. Problems can arise when discussions meander from clinical topics, however. Because front-line agency work can be very stressful, workers often feel the need to complain about organizational problems. It is helpful if a clear ground rule is established early on that only clinical case material or multisystemic case issues will be discussed during this time. It is also helpful to rotate presentations so that all members of the group have an opportunity to benefit from the peer supervisory process.

Training as an Antidote to Burnout

Boyd-Franklin (1989) discusses regular staff training as an "antidote to burnout." Supervision often provides a direct "lifeline" for family workers. Ongoing training offers an opportunity for all workers to keep their skills current and developed. Recent developments in the field, such as the impact of managed care and the funding priorities of state and national agencies, are appropriate topics for training. Special topics and current developments in various areas (cultural competency, cross-racial treatment, drug and alcohol dependency, physical abuse and neglect, sexual abuse, domestic violence, gang violence, etc.) can be offered. It is not always necessary to go outside an agency to find speakers. Senior staff members with expertise in a particular area can feel very empowered if they are invited to give presentations to the rest of their colleagues. Also, since few agencies have budgets extensive enough to send all staff members to professional conferences, one staff person can attend the conference with the understanding that he or she will then do in-service training for other staff members. It is helpful if this responsibility is rotated so that everyone benefits.

Professional Growth and Development

Another casualty of cost cutting has been a decrease in ongoing attention to the professional growth and development of staff members. This is a major loss, because these discussions can also serve as an antidote to burnout. Successful supervisors and administrators often make the time to discuss professional development plans with each staff member at least once per year. This support, although minimal in time, has many benefits in terms of staff morale and energy. Regular discussion of continuing education programs being offered by professional organizations can provide an incentive for further growth and training. Although few agencies can afford to pay for this training, this is a situation where a "comp time" arrangement is appropriate: Staff members can arrange with their senior administrator to work additional hours in order to be allowed to attend a training activity.

Career plans and further education can also be discussed with supervisees. Sometimes these goals must be conceived of as "long-term" since they might constitute "overload" in a trainee's current situation. It is important that future plans be discussed individually in a supportive atmosphere, and that all staff members have the benefit of this encouragement, not just the "chosen few."

Audio- and Videotaping

It is, of course, ideal from a supervisory point of view to have audiotapes or videotapes of sessions available on a regular basis. Because it can often be difficult to carry cumbersome equipment to home-based sessions, agencies may consider purchasing camcorders (small video cameras) or small tape recorders that can be rotated among staff members.

With some clients and family members, however, particularly those who have had encounters with the police or are mandated by the courts to seek therapy, taping may be reminiscent of the arrest process and can lead to suspicion and resistance. In addition, African American and other ethnic minority families, having had years of experience with racism and discrimination, often mistrust agencies (see Chapters 2 and 8). Members of such families may initially refuse audiotaping or videotaping until trust has been established with the family worker. Family workers who have encountered resistance when this topic is first raised should be encouraged to raise it again after trust has been established.

There are various ways in which this issue may be presented by the family worker. Here is one example: "When the entire family meets together, things happen too quickly for me to be able to remember everything each of you says. I would like to be able to hear everything and think about it between meetings." Such a statement serves two purposes: (1) It acknowledges the family worker's interest in the contribution of each family member, and (2) it conveys to the family members that the worker thinks about them between sessions. Another approach might be as follows: "Because I do home-based work, I'm in my car driving around a great deal. It is very helpful to have a tape that I can listen to while I'm driving, so that I can process important issues and come up with ideas that can be helpful to you."

If the worker would like to use the tape for supervision and has shared with the family that he or she has a supervisor, it may be helpful in some instances to say, "As you know, every worker in our agency has a supervisor, who works with us to brainstorm solutions for our families. It would be a big help if I could share with her [him] an audiotape [or videotape] of a session so that he [she] has more of a sense of who you are." Once again, the worker should be careful to present this matter-of-factly and to avoid presenting supervision as a hierarchical, one-down relationship. This can result in the worker's loss of credibility and power within the therapeutic relationship. In this situation, clients often speak directly to the supervisor when sessions are being taped. This clearly should be avoided.

In cases where a multidisciplinary team or case conference approach is used, this can be presented to the family as follows: "One of the benefits about working with our agency is that we use a team approach. That means we can have the input of our coworkers whenever you want it. This is a particularly crucial time for you, and it may be helpful to get their input. Since I can't bring them out to you, we can audiotape or videotape a session and I will bring back their comments."

Finally, if resistance to the taping process continues, the worker should respect the family's wishes and boundaries. When a family firmly says "no," repeatedly pushing harder is often not helpful (Kagan & Schlossberg, 1989). In these circumstances, family workers, particularly those who are seeing a number of families in the course of the day, are encouraged to carry a notebook with them and to write down key points after each session.

EMPOWERMENT OF FAMILY THERAPISTS
AND SUPERVISORS

As we have stated throughout this book, our primary goal is *to empower families, family therapists, and their supervisors.* We believe that isolation is a major problem for families and for family therapists. Therefore we encourage all supervisors and family therapists to use training conferences and agency outreach, as well as in-house case conferences, as an opportunity to build support networks for themselves. This work is very exciting and challenging, but it can also be very difficult and demanding at times. It is crucial that family therapists find peer networks and supervision that can sustain them in this work. It is our hope that this book has also provided a knowledge base that will empower family therapists and supervisors to do their jobs even more effectively.

References

Alexander, A. S. (1997). *The impact of behavioral family therapy on early adolescent problems: Replication and an attempt to enhance outcome through neighborhood parent meetings.* Unpublished master's thesis, Rutgers University.

Alexander, P. (1990). Intervention with incestuous families. In S. W. Henggeler & C. M. Borduin (Eds.), *Family therapy and beyond: A multisystemic approach to treating the behavior problems of children and adolescents* (pp. 324–344). Pacific Grove, CA: Brooks/Cole.

Allen, J. P., Leadbeater, B. J., & Aber, J. L. (1994). The development of problem behavior syndromes in at-risk adolescents. *Development and Psychopathology, 6,* 323–342.

Aponte, H. (1976). Underorganization in the poor family. In P. J. Guerin (Ed.), *Family therapy: Theory and practice* (pp. 432–438). New York: Gardner Press.

Aponte, H. (1985). The negotiation of values in therapy. *Family Process, 24*(3), 323–338.

Aponte, H. (1995). *Bread and spirit: Therapy with the new poor.* New York: Norton.

Bailey, S. L., Flewelling, R. L., & Rachal, J. V. (1992). Predicting continued use of marijuana among adolescents: The relative influence of drug-specific and social context factors. *Journal of Health and Social Behavior, 33,* 51–66.

Barkley, R. A. (1995). *Taking charge of ADHD: The complete, authoritative guide for parents.* New York: Guilford Press.

Barkley, R. A. (1998). *Attention-deficit hyperactivity disorder: A handbook for diagnosis and treatment* (2nd ed.). New York: Guilford Press.

Barnes, G. M., & Welte, J. W. (1990). Prediction of adults' drinking patterns from the drinking of their parents. *Journal of Studies on Alcohol, 51,* 523–527.

Barnett, W. S., & Escobar, C. M. (1990). Economic costs and benefits of early intervention. In S. J. Meisels & J. P. Shonkoff (Eds.), *Handbook of early childhood intervention* (pp. 560–582). New York: Cambridge University Press.

Beier, J. J. (1990). *Adolescent verbal behavior associated with reported substance use and substance refusal.* Unpublished doctoral dissertation, Rutgers University.

Belle, D. (1990). Poverty and women's mental health. *American Psychologist,* 45(3), 385–389.

Bennett, M. E. (1995). *Predictors of continuity of problem drinking from young adulthood to adulthood.* Unpublished doctoral dissertation, Rutgers University.

Benson, C. S., & Heller, K. (1987). Factors in the current adjustment of young adult daughters of alcoholic and problem drinking fathers. *Journal of Abnormal Psychology, 96,* 305–312.

Berg, I. K. (1994). *Family based services: A solution-focused approach.* New York: Norton.

Bernal, G. (1982). Cuban families. In M. McGoldrick, J. K. Pearce, & J. Giordano (Eds.), *Ethnicity and family therapy* (pp. 187–207). New York: Guilford Press.

Bernal, G., & Gutierrez, M. (1988). Cubans. In L. Comas-Díaz & E. E. H. Griffiths (Eds.), *Clinical guidelines in cross-cultural mental health* (pp. 233–261). New York: Wiley.

Bernal, G., & Shapiro, E. (1996). Cuban families. In M. McGoldrick, J. Giordano, & J. K. Pearce (Eds.), *Ethnicity and family therapy* (2nd ed., pp. 155–168). New York: Guilford Press.

Berrueta-Clement, J. R., Schweinhart, L. J., Barnett, W. S., & Weikart, D. P. (1987). The effects of early educational intervention on crime and delinquency in adolescence and early adulthood. In J. D. Burchard & S. N. Burchard (Eds.), *Prevention of delinquent behavior* (pp. 220–240). Beverly Hills, CA: Sage.

Biglan, A. (1995). *Changing cultural practices: A contextualist framework for intervention research.* Reno, NV: Context Press.

Billingsley, A. (1968). *Black families in White America.* Englewood Cliffs, NJ: Prentice-Hall.

Billingsley, A. (1992). *Climbing Jacob's ladder: The enduring legacy of African-American families.* New York: Simon & Schuster.

Black, M. M., & Krishnakumar, A. (1998). Children in low-income, urban settings: Interventions to promote mental health and well-being. *American Psychologist, 53,* 635–646.

Blechman, E. A. (1985). *Solving child behavior problems at home and at school.* Champaign, IL: Research Press.

Block, J., Block, J. H., & Keyes, S. (1988). Longitudinally foretelling drug usage in adolescence: Early childhood personality and environmental precursors. *Child Development, 59,* 336–355.

Borduin, C. M., Mann, B. T., Cone, L. T., Henggeler, S. W., Fucci, B. R., Blaske, D. M., & Williams, R. A. (1995). Multisystemic treatment of serious juvenile offenders: Long-term prevention of criminality and violence. *Journal of Consulting and Clinical Psychology, 63,* 569–578.

Bowen, M. (1978). *Family therapy in clinical practice.* New York: Jason Aronson.

Boyd-Franklin, N. (1987). Group therapy for Black women: A therapeutic support model. *American Journal of Orthopsychiatry, 57*(3), 394–401.

Boyd-Franklin, N. (1989). *Black families in therapy: A multisystems approach.* New York: Guilford Press.

Boyd-Franklin, N. (1991). Recurrent themes in the treatment of Black women in group therapy. *Women and Therapy, 11*(2), 25–30.

Boyd-Franklin, N. (1993). Secrets in African-American families. In E. Imber-Black (Ed.), *Secrets in families and family therapy* (pp. 331–354). New York: Norton.

Boyd-Franklin, N. (1998). The application of a multisystems model to home and community based treatment of African American families. In R. Jones (Ed.), *African American mental health* (pp. 315–328). Hampton, VA: Cobb & Henry.

Boyd-Franklin, N., Aleman, J. D. C., Jean-Gilles, M. M., & Lewis, S. Y. (1995). Cultural sensitivity and competence: African-American, Latino, and Haitian families with HIV/AIDS. In N. Boyd-Franklin, G. L. Steiner, & M. G. Boland (Eds.), *Children, families, and HIV/AIDS: Psychosocial and therapeutic issues* (pp. 53–77). New York: Guilford Press.

Boyd-Franklin, N., & Franklin, A. J. (1998). African American couples in therapy. In M. McGoldrick (Ed.), *Re-visioning family therapy: Race, culture, and gender in clinical practice* (pp. 268–281). New York: Guilford Press.

Boyd-Franklin, N., Franklin, A. J., & Toussaint, P. (in press). *Boys to men: Raising our African American teenage sons.* New York: Dutton Press.

Boyd-Franklin, N., & Lockwood, T. W. (1999). Spirituality and religion: Implications for psychotherapy with African American clients and families. In F. Walsh (Ed.), *Spiritual resources in family therapy* (pp. 90–103). New York: Guilford Press.

Boyd-Franklin, N., Morris, T. S., & Bry, B. (1997). Parent and family support groups with African American families: The process of community empowerment. *Cultural Diversity and Mental Health, 3*(2), 83–92.

Boyd-Franklin, N., Steiner, G. L., & Boland, M. G. (Eds.). (1995). *Children, families, and HIV/AIDS: Psychosocial and therapeutic issues.* New York: Guilford Press.

Brazelton, T. B. (1972). *Infants and mothers: Differences in development.* New York: Dell.

Briere, J. (1988). The long-term clinical correlates of childhood sexual victimization. *Annals of the New York Academy of Sciences, 528,* 327–334.

Briere, J., & Zaidi, L. Y. (1989). Sexual abuse histories and sequelae in female psychiatric emergency room patients. *American Journal of Psychiatry, 146*(12), 1602–1606.

Bronfenbrenner, U. (1979). *The ecology of human development: Experiments by nature and design.* Cambridge, MA: Harvard University.

Bronfenbrenner, U., & Weiss, H. (1983). Beyond policies without people: An ecological perspective on child and family policy. In S. Kagan, E. Klugman, & E. Zigler (Eds.), *Children, families, and government* (pp. 393–414). Cambridge, MA: Cambridge University Press.

Brook, J. S. (1993). Interactional theory: Its utility in explaining drug use behavior among African-American and Puerto Rican youth. In M. R. De La Rosa & J.-L. Recio Adrados (Eds.), *Drug abuse among minority youth: Advances in research and methodology* (NIDA Research Monograph No. 130, pp. 79–101). Rockville, MD: National Institute on Drug Abuse.

Brook, J. S., Brook, D. W., Gordon, A. S., Whiteman, M., & Cohen, P. (1990). The psychosocial etiology of adolescent drug use: A family interactional approach. *Genetic, Social, and General Psychology Monographs, 116*(2), 111–267.

Brook, J. S., Whiteman, M., Cohen, P., & Tanaka, J. S. (1991). Childhood precursors of adolescent's drug use: A longitudinal analysis. *Genetic, Social, and General Psychology Monographs, 118*(2), 195–213.

Brook, J. S., Whiteman, M., Gordon, A. S., & Brook, D. W. (1984). Paternal determinants of female adolescent's marijuana use. *Developmental Psychology, 20*(6), 1032–1043.

Brunswick, A., Messeri, P., & Titus, S. (1992). Predictive factors in adult substance abuse: A prospective study of African American adolescents. In M. Glantz & R. Pickens (Eds.), *Vulnerability to drug abuse* (pp. 419–464). Washington, DC: American Psychological Association.

Bry, B. H. (1982). Reducing the incidence of adolescent problems through preventive intervention: One- and five-year follow-up. *American Journal of Community Psychology, 10*, 265–276.

Bry, B. H. (1994). Preventing substance abuse by supporting families' efforts with community resources. *Child & Family Behavior Therapy, 16*, 21–26.

Bry, B. H. (1996). Psychological approaches to prevention. In W. Bickel & R. DeGrandpre (Eds.), *Drug policy and human nature: Psychological perspectives on the prevention, management, and treatment of illicit drug use* (pp. 55–76). New York: Plenum Press.

Bry, B. H., & Alexander, A. S. (1997). Empirical foundations for using behavioral family therapy to prevent adolescent substance abuse. *The Family Psychologist, 13*(4), 12–13, 19, 22.

Bry, B. H., Conboy, C., & Bisgay, K. (1986). Decreasing adolescent drug use and school failure: Long-term effects of targeted family problem-solving training. *Child & Family Behavior Therapy, 8*, 43–59.

Bry, B. H., & George, F. E. (1980). The preventive effects of early intervention upon the attendance and grades of urban adolescents. *Professional Psychology, 11*, 252–260.

Bry, B. H., & Greene, D. M. (1988–1989). Providing family therapy through the schools. *Psychotherapy Bulletin, 23*(4), 21–23.

Bry, B. H., & Greene, D. M. (1990). Empirical bases for integrating school- and family-based interventions against early adolescent substance abuse. In R. McMahon & R. Peters (Eds.), *Behavior disorders of adolescence: Research, intervention, and policy in clinical and school settings* (pp. 81–97). New York: Plenum Press.

Bry, B. H., Greene, D. M., Schutte, C., & Fishman, C. A. (1991). *Targeted Family Intervention manual*. (Available from B. H. Bry, Graduate School of Applied and Professional Psychology, Rutgers University, 152 Frelinghuysen Road, Piscataway, NJ 08854-8085)

Bry, B. H., & Krinsley, K. E. (1990). Adolescent substance abuse: A case approach. In E. L. Feindler & G. R. Kalfus (Eds.), *Adolescent behavior therapy handbook* (pp. 275–302). New York: Springer.

Bry, B. H., & Krinsley, K. E. (1992). Booster sessions and long-term effects of behavioral family therapy on adolescent substance use and school performance. *Journal of Behavior Therapy and Experimental Psychiatry, 23*, 183–189.

Bry, B. H., McKeon, P., & Pandina, R. J. (1982). Extent of drug use as a function of number of risk factors. *Journal of Abnormal Psychology, 91*, 273–279.

Burnam, M. A., Stein, J. A., Golding, J. M., Siegel, J. M., Sorenson, S. B., Forsythe, A. B., & Telles, C. A. (1988). Sexual assault and mental disorders in a community population. *Journal of Consulting and Clinical Psychology, 56*(6), 843–850.

California State Council on Developmental Disabilities. (1989). *Program development fund cycle XE evaluation report*. Sacramento: Author.

Carter, R. T. (1990). Does race or racial identity attitudes influence the counseling process in Black–White dyads? In J. E. Helms (Ed.), *Black and White racial identity: Theory, research and practice* (pp. 145–163). Westport, CT: Greenwood Press.

Carter, R. T., & Helms, J. E. (1992). The counseling process as defined by relationship types: A test of Helm's interfactional model. *Journal of Multicultural Counseling and Development, 20*(4), 181–201.

Catalano, R. F., Hawkins, J. D., Krenz, C., Gillmore, M., Morrison, D., Wells, E., & Abbott, R. (1993). Using research to guide culturally appropriate drug abuse prevention. *Journal of Consulting and Clinical Psychology, 61*(5), 804–811.

Catalano, R. F., Morrison, D., Wells, E. A., Gillmore, M. R., Iritani, B., & Hawkins, J. D. (1992). Ethnic differences in family factors related to early drug initiation. *Journal of Studies on Alcohol, 53*(3), 208–217.

Chassin, L., Pillow, D., Curran, P., Molina, B., & Barrera, M. (1993). The relation of parent alcoholism to adolescent substance use: A test of three mediating mechanisms. *Journal of Abnormal Psychology, 102*, 3–19.

Chilcoat, H. D., Dishion, T. J., & Anthony, J. C. (1995). Parent monitoring and the incidence of drug sampling in urban elementary school children. *American Journal of Epidemiology, 141*, 25–31.

Christiansen, B. A., Goldman, M. S., & Brown, S. A. (1985). The differential development of adolescent alcohol expectancies may predict adult alcoholism. *Addictive Behaviors, 10*, 299–306.

Clark, L. (1985a). *SOS: Help for parents*. Bowling Green, KY: Parents Press.

Clark, L. (1985b). *SOS: Help for parents* [Videotape]. Bowling Green, KY: Parents Press.

Clayton, R. R. (1992). Transitions in drug use: Risk and protective factors. In M. Glantz & R. Pickens (Eds.), *Vulnerability to drug abuse* (pp. 15–51). Washington, DC: American Psychological Association.

Comas-Díaz, L., & Griffith, E. E. H. (Eds.). (1988). *Clinical guidelines in cross cultural mental health*. New York: Wiley.

Comer, J. P., & Hamilton-Lee, M. E. (1982). Support systems in the Black community. In D. E. Biegel & A. J. Naparstek (Eds.), *Community support systems and mental health* (pp. 121–136). New York: Springer.

Cotton, L., & Bynum, D. R. (1995, July). *The impact of socialization forces on the stability of work values from late adolescence to early adulthood*. Paper presented at the Seventh Annual Convention of the American Psychological Society, New York.

Crockenberg, S. B. (1981). Infant irritability, other responsiveness, and social support influences on the security of infant–mother attachment. *Child Development, 52,* 857–865.

Dattilio, F. M. (1998). Cognitive-behavioral family therapy. In F. M. Dattilio (Ed.), *Case studies in couple and family therapy: Systemic and cognitive perspectives* (pp. 62–84). New York: Guilford Press.

Dembo, R., Blount, W. R., Schmeidler, J., & Burgos, W. (1986). Perceived environmental drug use risk and the correlates of early drug use or nonuse among inner-city youths: The motivated actor. *International Journal of the Addictions, 21* (9–10), 977–1000.

Dembo, R., Williams, L., La Voie, L., Berry, E., Getreu, A., Wish, E. D., Schmeidler, J., & Washburn, M. (1989). Physical abuse, sexual victimization, and illicit drug use: Replication of a structural analysis among a new sample of high-risk youths. *Violence and Victims, 4*(2), 121–138.

Dembo, R., Williams, L., Wothke, W., Schmeidler, J., & Brown, C. H. (1992). The role of family factors, physical abuse, and sexual victimization experiences in high-risk youths' alcohol and other drug use and delinquency: A longitudinal model. *Violence and Victims, 7*(3), 245–266.

de Shazer, S. (1982). *Patterns of brief family therapy: An ecosystemic approach.* New York: Guilford Press.

Dishion, T. J., & Andrews, D. W. (1995). Preventing escalation in problem behaviors with high-risk young adolescents: Immediate and 1-year outcomes. *Journal of Consulting and Clinical Psychology, 63,* 538–548.

Dishion, T. J., & Patterson, S. G. (1996). *Preventive parenting with love, encouragement and limits: The preschool years.* Eugene, OR: Castalia.

Dishion, T. J., Reid, J. B., & Patterson, G. R. (1988). Empirical guidelines for a family intervention for adolescent drug use. *Journal of Chemical Dependency Treatment, 1*(2), 189–224.

Dornbusch, S. M., Ritter, P. L., Liederman, P., Roberts, D., & Fraleigh, M. (1987). The relation of parenting style to adolescent school performance. *Child Development, 58,* 1244–1257.

Dryfoos, J. G. (1990). *Adolescents at risk.* New York: Oxford University Press.

Dumas, J. E., Gibson, J. A., & Albin, J. B. (1989). Behavioral correlates of maternal depressive symptomatology in conduct-disorder children. *Journal of Consulting and Clinical Psychology, 57*(4), 516–521.

Dumas, J. E., LaFreniere, P. J., & Serketich, W. J. (1995). "Balance of power": A transactional analysis of control in mother–child dyads involving socially competent, aggressive, and anxious children. *Journal of Abnormal Psychology, 104*(1), 104–113.

Dumas, J. E., & Wahler, R. G. (1983). Predictors of treatment outcome in parent training: Mother insularity and socioeconomic disadvantage. *Behavioral Assessment, 5,* 301–313.

Duncan, T. E., Duncan, S. C., & Hops, H. (1994). The effects of family cohesiveness and peer encouragement on the development of adolescent alcohol use: A cohort-sequential approach to the analysis of longitudinal data. *Journal of Studies on Alcohol, 55*(5), 588–599.

D'Zurilla, T. J. (1986). *Problem-solving therapy: A social competence approach to clinical intervention*. New York: Springer.

El-Guebaly, N., & Offord, D. R. (1977). The offspring of alcoholics: A clinical review. *American Journal of Psychiatry, 134*, 357–365.

Ensminger, M. E. (1990). Sexual activity and problem behaviors among Black, urban adolescents. *Child Development, 61*, 2032–2046.

Eyberg, S. M. (1988). Parent–child interaction therapy: Integration of traditional and behavioral concerns. *Child & Family Behavior Therapy, 10*, 33–46.

Falicov, C. (1982). Mexican families. In M. McGoldrick, J. K. Pearce, & J. Giordano (Eds.), *Ethnicity and family therapy* (pp. 134–163). New York: Guilford Press.

Falicov, C. (1996). Mexican families. In M. McGoldrick, J. Giordano, & J. K. Pearce (Eds.), *Ethnicity and family therapy* (2nd ed., pp. 169–182). New York: Guilford Press.

Falicov, C. (1998). *Latino families in therapy: A guide to multicultural practice*. New York: Guilford Press.

Falloon, I. R. H. (1991). Behavioral family therapy. In A. S. Gurman & D. P. Kniskern (Eds.), *Handbook of family therapy, Vol. II* (pp. 65–95). New York: Brunner/Mazel.

Farrell, A. D., & White, K. S. (1998). Peer influences and drug use among urban adolescents: Family structure and parent–adolescent relationship as protective factors. *Journal of Consulting and Clinical Psychology, 66*, 248–258.

Finkelhor, D. (1995). The victimization of children: A developmental perspective. *American Journal of Orthopsychiatry, 65*(2), 177–193.

Finkelhor, D., & Dziuba-Leatherman, J. (1994). Victimization of children. *American Psychologist, 49*(3), 173–183.

Fitzgerald, H. E., Sullivan, L. A., Ham, H. P., Zucker, R. A., Bruckel, S., Schneider, A. M., & Noll, R. B. (1993). Predictors of behavior problems in three-year-old sons of alcoholics: Early evidence for the onset of risk. *Child Development, 64*, 110–123.

Forehand, R. L., & McMahon, R. J. (1981). *Helping the noncompliant child: A clinician's guide to parent training*. New York: Guilford Press.

Forehand, R., Miller, K. S., Dutra, R., & Chance, M. W. (1997). Role of parenting in adolescent deviant behavior: Replication across and within ethnic groups. *Journal of Consulting and Clinical Psychology, 65*, 1036–1041.

Franklin, A. J. (1993, July–August). The invisibility syndrome. *Family Therapy Networker*, pp. 33–39.

Frazier, E. F. (1963). *The negro church in America*. New York: Schocken.

Furstenberg, F. F., Brooks-Gunn, J., & Morgan, S. P. (1987). *Adolescent mothers in later life*. Cambridge, UK: Cambridge University Press.

Garcia, J. G., & Zea, M. C. (Eds.). (1997). *Psychological interventions and research with Latino populations*. Needham Heights, MA: Allyn & Bacon.

Garcia-Preto, N. (1996). Latino families: An overview. In M. McGoldrick, J. Giordano, & J. K. Pearce (Eds.), *Ethnicity and family therapy* (2nd ed., pp. 141–154). New York: Guilford Press.

Gardere, J. (1999). *Smart parenting for African Americans: Helping your kids thrive in a difficult world.* Secaucus, NJ: Citadel Press.

Gibbs, J. T. (1998). African American adolescents. In J. T. Gibbs & L. N. Huang (Eds.), *Children of color: Psychological interventions with culturally diverse youth* (pp. 171–214). San Francisco: Jossey-Bass.

Gibbs, J. T., & Huang, L. N. (Eds.). (1998). *Children of color: Psychological interventions with culturally diverse youth.* San Francisco: Jossey-Bass.

Gil, E. (1994). *Play in family therapy.* New York: Guilford Press.

Gil, E. (1995). *Systemic treatment of families who abuse.* San Francisco: Jossey-Bass.

Gil, E. (1996). *Treating abused adolescents.* New York: Guilford Press.

Gottfredson, M. R., & Hirschi, T. (1994). A general theory of adolescent problem behavior: Problems and prospects. In R. D. Ketterlinus & M. E. Lamb (Eds.), *Adolescent problem behaviors: Issues and research* (pp. 41–56). Hillsdale, NJ: Erlbaum.

Greene, D. M., & Bry, B. H. (1991). A descriptive analysis of family discussions about everyday problems and decisions. *The Analysis of Verbal Behavior, 9,* 29–39.

Grier, W., & Cobbs, P. (1968). *Black rage.* New York: Basic Books.

Haley, J. (1976). *Problem-solving therapy.* San Francisco: Jossey-Bass.

Hardy, K. V. (1989). The theoretical myth of sameness: A critical issue in family therapy training and treatment. *Journal of Psychotherapy and the Family, 6*(1–2), 17–33.

Hartman, A., & Laird, J. (1983). *Family-centered social work practice.* New York: Free Press.

Hawkins, J. D., Catalano, R. F., & Associates. (1992). *Communities that care.* San Francisco: Jossey-Bass.

Hawkins, J. D., Catalano, R. F., Morrison, D. M., O'Donnell, J., Abbott, R. D., & Day, L. E. (1992). The Seattle social development project: Effects of the first four years on protective factors and problem behaviors. In J. McCord & R. E. Tremblay (Eds.), *Preventing antisocial behavior: Interventions from birth through adolescence* (pp. 139–161). New York: Guilford Press.

Hawkins, J. D., Von Cleve, E., & Catalano, R. F. (1991). Reducing early childhood aggression: Results of a primary prevention program. *Journal of the American Academy of Child and Adolescent Psychiatry, 30,* 208–217.

Helms, J. E., & Cook, D. A. (1999). *Using race and culture in counseling and psychotherapy: Theory and process.* Needham Heights, MA: Allyn & Bacon.

Hendin, H., Pollinger, A., Ulman, R., & Carr, A. C. (1981). *Adolescent marijuana abusers and their families* (NIDA Research Monograph No. 40). Rockville, MD: National Institute on Drug Abuse.

Henggeler, S. W., & Borduin, C. M. (Eds.). (1990). *Family therapy and beyond: A multisystemic approach to treating the behavior problems of children and adolescents.* Pacific Grove, CA: Brooks/Cole.

Henggeler, S. W., Melton, G. B., Brondino, M. J., Schere, D. G., & Hanley, J. H. (1997). Multisystemic therapy with violent and chronic juvenile offenders and their families: The role of treatment fidelity in successful dissemination. *Journal of Consulting and Clinical Psychology, 65,* 821–833.

Henggeler, S. W., Melton, G. B., & Smith, L. A. (1992). Family preservation using multisystemic therapy: An effective alternative to incarcerating serious juvenile offenders. *Journal of Consulting and Clinical Psychology, 60,* 953–961.

Henggeler, S. W., Pickrel, S. G., Brondino, M. J., & Crouch, J. L. (1996). Eliminating (almost) treatment dropout of substance abusing or dependent delinquents through home-based multisystemic therapy. *American Journal of Psychiatry, 15,* 427–428.

Henggeler, S. W., Schoenwald, S. K., Borduin, C. M., Rowland, M. D., & Cunningham, P. B. (1998). *Multisystemic treatment of antisocial behavior in children and adolescents.* New York: Guilford Press.

Hill, R. (1972). *The strengths of Black families.* New York: Emerson-Hall.

Hines, P. M., & Boyd-Franklin, N. (1982). Black families. In M. McGoldrick, J. K. Pearce, & J. Giordano (Eds.), *Ethnicity and family therapy* (pp. 84–107). New York: Guilford Press.

Hines, P. M., & Boyd-Franklin, N. (1996). African American families. In M. McGoldrick, J. Giordano, & J. K. Pearce (Eds.), *Ethnicity and family therapy* (2nd. ed., pp. 66–84). New York: Guilford Press.

Hunt, P. (1987). Black clients: Implications for supervision of trainees. *Psychotherapy, 24*(1), 114–119.

Imber-Black, E. (Ed.). (1993). *Secrets in families and family therapy.* New York: Norton.

Inclan, J. E., & Herron, D. G. (1998). Puerto Rican adolescents. In J. T. Gibbs & L. N. Huang (Eds.), *Children of color: Psychological interventions with culturally diverse youth* (pp. 240–263). San Francisco: Jossey-Bass.

Itzkowitz, A. (1989). Children in placement: A place for family therapy. In L. Combrinck-Graham (Ed.), *Children in family contexts: Perspectives on treatment* (pp. 391–412). New York: Guilford Press.

Jacobson, N. S. (1984). A component analysis of behavior marital therapy: The relative effectiveness of behavior exchange and communication problem solving. *Journal of Consulting and Clinical Psychology, 52,* 295–305.

Jaffe, P., Wolfe, D., Wilson, S., & Zak, L. (1986). Similarities in behavioral and social maladjustment among child victims and witnesses to family violence. *American Journal of Orthopsychiatry, 56*(1), 142–146.

Jansen, R. E., Fitzgerald, H. E., Ham, H. P., & Zucker, R. A. (1995). Pathways into risk: Temperament and behavior problems in three- to five-year-old sons of alcoholics. *Alcoholism: Clinical and Experimental Research, 19*(2), 501–509.

Jessor, R., & Jessor, S. L. (1977). *Problem behavior and psychosocial development: A longitudinal study of youth.* New York: Academic Press.

Johnson, H. L., Glassman, M. B., Fiks, K. B., & Rosen, T. S. (1990). Resilient children: Individual differences in developmental outcome of children born to drug abusers. *Journal of Genetic Psychology, 151*(4), 523–539.

Johnson, V., & Pandina, R. J. (1991). Effects of the family environment on adolescent substance use, delinquency, and coping styles. *American Journal of Drug and Alcohol Abuse, 17*(1), 71–88.

Jones, D. C., & Houts, R. (1992). Parental drinking, parent–child communication, and social skills in young adults. *Journal of Studies on Alcohol, 53*(1), 48–56.

Jones, R. L. (Ed.). (1988). *Psychoeducational assessment of minority group children: A casebook*. Hampton, VA: Cobbs & Henry.

Kagan, R., & Schlossberg, S. (1989). *Families in perpetual crisis*. New York: Norton.

Kagan, S., Powell, D., Weissbourd, B., & Zigler, E. (Eds.). (1987). *America's family support programs*. New Haven, CT: Yale University Press.

Kandel, D. B., & Davies, M. (1992). Progression to regular marijuana involvement: Phenomenology and risk factors for near-daily use. In M. Glantz & R. Pickens (Eds.), *Vulnerability to drug abuse* (pp. 211–242). Washington, DC: American Psychological Association.

Kandel, D. B., Kessler, R. C., & Margulies, R. Z. (1978). Adolescent initiation into stages of drug use: A developmental analysis. In D. B. Kandel (Ed.), *Longitudinal research on drug use: Empirical findings and methodological issues* (pp. 73–99). Washington, DC: Hemisphere–Wiley.

Kaplan, H. B., & Johnson, R. J. (1992). Relationships between circumstances surrounding initial illicit drug use and escalation of drug use: Moderating effects of gender and early adolescent experiences. In M. Glantz & R. Pickens (Eds.), *Vulnerability to drug abuse* (pp. 299–352). Washington, DC: American Psychological Association.

Kavanagh, K. A., Youngblade, L., Reid, J. B., & Fagot, B. I. (1988). Interactions between children and abusive versus control parents. *Journal of Clinical Child Psychology, 17*(2), 137–142.

Kellam, S. G., Brown, C. H., Rubin, B. R., & Ensminger, M. E. (1983). Paths leading to teenage psychiatric symptoms and substance use: Developmental epidemiological studies in Woodlawn. In S. B. Guze, F. J. Earls, & J. E. Barrett (Eds.), *Childhood psychopathology and development* (pp. 17–51). New York: Raven Press.

Krinsley, K. E. (1991). Behavioral family therapy for adolescent school problems: School performance effects and generalization to substance use (Doctoral dissertation, Rutgers University, 1991). *Dissertation Abstracts International, 52*, 1725B.

Krinsley, K. E., & Bry, B. H. (1992). Sequential analyses of adolescent, mother, and father behaviors in distressed and nondistressed families. *Child & Family Behavior Therapy, 13*, 45–62.

Krohn, M. D., & Thornberry, T. P. (1993). Network theory: A model for understanding drug abuse among African-American and Hispanic youth. In M. R. De La Rosa & J. L. Recio Adrados (Eds.), *Drug abuse among minority youth: Advances in research and methodology* (NIDA Research Monograph No. 130, pp. 102–128). Rockville, MD: National Institute on Drug Abuse.

Kumpfer, K. L. (1990). Environmental and family-focused prevention: The Cinderellas of prevention want to go to the ball, too. In K. H. Rey, C. L. Faegre, & P. Lowery (Eds.), *Prevention research findings: 1988* (OSAP Prevention Monograph No. 3, DHHS Publication No. ADM 89-1615, pp. 194–220). Washington, DC: U.S. Government Printing Office.

Kumpfer, K. L., & DeMarsh, J. P. (1986). Family-oriented interventions for the prevention of chemical dependency in children and adolescents. In S. Griswold-Ezekoye, K. L. Kumpfer, & W. Bukoski (Eds.), *Childhood and chemical abuse: Prevention and intervention* (pp. 49–91). New York: Haworth Press.

Kunjufu, J. (1985). *Countering the conspiracy to destroy Black boys.* Chicago: African-American Images.

Lang, A. R. (1992). Parental drinking and child behavior problems: A case of bidirectional influences? *the Behavior Therapist, 15*(1), 15–17.

Lee, E. (1996). Asian American families: An overview. In M. McGoldrick, J. Giordano, & J. K. Pearce (Eds.), *Ethnicity and family therapy* (2nd ed., pp. 227–248). New York: Guilford Press.

Liddle, H. A., Dakof, G. A., & Diamond, G. (1991). Adolescent substance abuse: Multidimensional family therapy in action. In E. Kaufman & P. Kaufmann (Eds.), *Family therapy approaches with drug and alcohol problems* (2nd ed.). Needham Heights, MA: Allyn & Bacon.

Lindahl, K. M. (1998). Family process variables and children's disruptive behavior problems. *Journal of Family Psychology, 12,* 420–436.

Lindblad-Goldberg, M., Dore, M. M., & Stern, L. (1998). *Creating competence from chaos: A comprehensive guide to home-based services.* New York: Norton.

Loeber, R. (1990). Development and risk factors of juvenile antisocial behavior and delinquency. *Clinical Psychology Review, 10,* 1–41.

Lutzker, J. R., Campbell, R. V., Newman, M. R., & Harrold, M. (1989). Ecobehavioral interventions for abusive, neglectful, and high-risk families. In G. H. S. Singer & L. K. Irvin (Eds.), *Support for caregiving families enabling positive adaptation to disability* (pp. 313–326). Baltimore: Paul H. Brookes.

Lutzker, J. R., & Rice, J. M. (1987). Using recidivism data to evaluate Project 12-Ways: An ecobehavioral approach to the treatment and prevention of child abuse and neglect. *Journal of Family Violence, 2*(4), 283–290.

MacFarlane, K., Waterman, J., Conerly, S., Damon, L., Durfee, M., & Long, S. (1986). *Sexual abuse of young children: Evaluation and treatment.* New York: Guilford Press.

Mansheim, P. A. (1989). The family in the legal system: The family turned against itself. In L. Combrinck-Graham (Ed.), *Children in family contexts: Perspectives on treatment* (pp. 369–390). New York: Guilford Press.

McAdoo, H. P. (Ed.). (1981). *Black families.* Beverly Hills, CA: Sage.

McAdoo, H. P., & McAdoo, J. L. (Eds.). (1985). *Black children: Social, educational and parental environments.* Beverly Hills, CA: Sage.

McCrady, B. S., & Epstein, E. E. (1995). Marital therapy in the treatment of alcohol problems. In N. S. Jacobson & A. S. Gurman (Eds.), *Clinical handbook of couple therapy* (pp. 369–393). New York: Guilford Press.

McGoldrick, M., & Gerson, R. (1985). *Genograms in family assessment.* New York: Norton.

McGoldrick, M., Gerson, R., & Shellenberger, S. (1999). *Genograms: Assessment and intervention* (2nd ed.). New York: Norton.

McGoldrick, M., Giordano, J., & Pearce, J. K. (Eds.). (1996). *Ethnicity and family therapy* (2nd ed.). New York: Guilford Press.

McGoldrick, M., Pearce, J. K., & Giordano, J. (Eds.). (1982). *Ethnicity and family therapy.* New York: Guilford Press.

Miller, B. A., Downs, W. R., Gondoli, D. M., & Keil, A. V. (1987). Childhood sexual abuse incidents for alcoholic women versus a random household sample. *Violence and Victims, 2*, 157–172.

Miller, D. (1989). Family violence and the helping system. In L. Combrinck-Graham (Ed.), *Children in family contexts: Perspectives on treatment* (pp. 413–436). New York: Guilford Press.

Minuchin, S. (1974). *Families and family therapy.* Cambridge, MA: Harvard University Press.

Minuchin, S., & Fishman, H. C. (1981). *Family therapy techniques.* Cambridge, MA: Harvard University Press.

Minuchin, S., & Nichols, M. (1993). *Family healing: Tales of hope and renewal from family therapy.* New York: Free Press.

Mitchell, H., & Lewter, N. (1986). *Soul theology: The heart of American Black culture.* San Francisco: Harper & Row.

Munger, R. L. (1993). *Changing children's behavior quickly.* Lanham, MD: Madison.

Muñoz, R. F., Snowden, L. R., & Kelly, J. G. (1979). *Social and psychological research in community settings.* San Francisco: Jossey-Bass.

National Research Council. (1993). *Losing generations: Adolescents in high-risk settings.* Washington, DC: National Academy Press.

Newcomb, M. D. (1988). *Drug use in the workplace: Risk factors for disruptive substance use among young adults.* Dover, MA: Auburn House.

Newcomb, M. D., Huba, G. J., & Bentler, P. M. (1983). Mother's influence on the drug use of their children: Confirmatory test of direct modeling and mediational theories. *Developmental Psychology, 19*(5), 714–726.

Nobles, W. (1980). African philosophy: Foundations for Black psychology. In R. Jones (Ed.). *Black psychology* (2nd ed., pp. 23–36). New York: Harper & Row.

Nye, C. L., Zucker, R. A., & Fitzgerald, H. E. (1995). Early intervention in the path to alcohol problems through conduct problems: Treatment involvement and child behavior change. *Journal of Consulting and Clinical Psychology, 63*(5), 831–840.

Office of Technology Assessment. (1990). *Indian adolescent mental health* (Report No. OTA-H-446). Washington, DC: U.S. Government Printing Office.

Parece, R. L. (1997). *Patterns of daily hassles and their appraisal in low income single mothers: Effects of information on prevention workers.* Unpublished doctoral dissertation, Rutgers University.

Parker, M. A. (1995). *Casual statements of families with adolescent problems.* Unpublished master's thesis, Rutgers University.

Patterson, G. R. (1995). Coercion as a basis for early age of onset for arrest. In J. McCord (Ed.), *Coercion and punishment in long-term perspectives* (pp. 81–105). Cambridge, UK: Cambridge University Press.

Patterson, G. R., & Forgatch, M. S. (1987). *Parents and adolescents living together: Vol. 1. The basics.* Eugene, OR: Castalia.

Patterson, G. R., & Forgatch, M. S. (1990). Initiation and maintenance of process disrupting single-mother families. In G. Patterson (Ed.), *Depression and aggression in family interaction* (pp. 209–245). Hillsdale, NJ: Erlbaum.

Patterson, G. R., Reid, J. B., Jones, R. R., & Conger, R. E. (1975). *A social learning approach to family intervention* (Vol. 1). Eugene, OR: Castalia.

Pizzo, P. (1983). *Parent to parent: Working together for ourselves and our children.* Boston: Beacon Press.

Pizzo, P. (1987). Parent-to-parent support groups: Advocates for social change. In S. Kagan, D. Powell, B. Weissbourd, & E. Zigler (Eds.), *America's family support programs* (pp. 161–181). New Haven, CT: Yale University Press.

Pollack, G. H. (1970). Anniversary reactions: Trauma and mourning. *Psychoanalytic Quarterly, 39,* 347–371.

Polusny, M. A., & Follette, V. M. (1995). Long-term correlates of child sexual abuse: Theory and review of the empirical literature. *Applied and Preventive Psychology, 4,* 143–166.

Ramirez, O. (1998). Mexican American children and adolescents. In J. T. Gibbs & L. N. Huang (Eds.), *Children of color: Psychological interventions with culturally diverse youth* (pp. 215–239). San Francisco: Jossey-Bass.

Rappaport, J. (1987). Terms of empowerment/exemplars of prevention: Toward a theory of community psychology. *American Journal of Community Psychology, 15*(2), 121–143.

Rhodes, J. E., Contreras, J. M., & Mangelsdorf, S. C. (1994). Natural mentor relationships among Latina adolescent mothers: Psychological adjustment, moderating processes, and the role of early parental acceptance. *American Journal of Community Psychology, 22*(2), 211–227.

Rhodes, J. E., Ebert, L., & Fischer, K. (1992). Natural mentors: An overlooked resource in the social networks of African-American adolescent mothers. *American Journal of Community Psychology, 20,* 445–462.

Richardson, J. L., Dwyer, K., McGuigan, K., Hansen, W. B., Dent, C., Johnson, C. A., Sussman, S. Y., Brannon, B., & Flay, B. (1989). Substance use among eighth-grade students who take care of themselves after school. *Pediatrics, 84*(3), 556–566.

Rickel, A. U., & Becker, E. (1997). *Keeping children from harm's way: How national policy affects psychological development.* Washington, DC: American Psychological Association.

Rigsby, L. C., Stull, J. C., & Morse-Kelley, N. (1997). Determinants of student educational expectations and achievement: Race/ethnicity and gender differences. In R. D. Taylor & M. C. Wang (Eds.), *Social and emotional adjustment and family relations in ethnic minority families* (pp. 201–223). Mahwah, NJ: Erlbaum.

Robin, A. L., & Foster, S. L. (1989). *Negotiating parent–adolescent conflict: A behavioral–family systems approach.* New York: Guilford Press.

Robins, L. N., & Przybeck, T. R. (1985). Age of onset of drug use as a factor in drug and other disorders. In C. L. Jones & R. J. Battjes (Eds.), *Etiology of drug abuse: Implications for prevention* (NIDA Research Monograph No. 56, pp. 178–192). Rockville, MD: National Institute on Drug Abuse.

Rodick, J. D., & Henggeler, S. W. (1980). The short-term and long-term amelioration of academic and motivational deficiencies among low-achieving inner-city adolescents. *Child Development, 51,* 1126–1132.

Rohsenow, D., Corbett, R., & Devine, D. (1988). Molested as children: A hidden contribution to substance abuse? *Journal of Substance Abuse Treatment, 5,* 13–18.

Sanders, M. R., & Dadds, M. R. (1993). *Behavioral family intervention.* Needham Heights, MA: Allyn & Bacon.

Schmidt, S. E., Liddle, H. A., & Dakof, G. (1996). Changes in parenting practices and adolescent drug abuse during multidimensional family therapy. *Journal of Family Psychology, 10,* 12–27.

Schorr, L. B. (1997). *Common purpose: Strengthening families and neighborhoods to rebuild America.* New York: Anchor Books.

Seitz, V. (1990). Intervention programs for impoverished children: A comparison of educational and family support models. *Annals of Child Development, 7,* 73–103.

Seitz, V., Rosenbaum, L. K., & Apfel, N. H. (1985). Effects of family support intervention: A ten-year follow-up. *Child Development, 53,* 376–391.

Seligman, M. E. P. (1990). *Learned optimism.* New York: Pocket Books.

Senchak, M., Leonard, K. E., Greene, B. W., & Carroll, A. (1995). Comparisons of adult children of alcoholic, divorced, and control parents in four outcome domains. *Psychology of Addictive Behaviors, 9*(3), 147–156.

Shedler, J., & Block, J. (1990). Adolescent drug use and psychological health: A longitudinal inquiry. *American Psychologist, 45*(5), 612–630.

Sher, K. J., Walitzer, K. S., Wood, P. K., & Brent, E. E. (1991). Characteristics of children of alcoholics: Putative risk factors, substance use and abuse, and psychopathology. *Journal of Abnormal Psychology, 100*(4), 427–448.

Shure, M. B., & Spivack, G. (1988). Interpersonal cognitive problem solving. In R. H. Price, E. L. Cowen, R. P. Lorion, & J. Ramos-McKay (Eds.), *Fourteen ounces of prevention* (pp. 69–82). Hyattsville, MD: American Psychological Association.

Slattery, M., Alderson, M. R., & Bryant, J. S. (1986). The occupational risks of alcoholism. *International Journal of the Addictions, 21*(8), 929–936.

Smart, R. G., & Gray, G. (1979). Parental and peer influences as correlates of problem drinking among high school students. *International Journal of the Addictions, 14*(7), 905–917.

Smith, C., Lizotte, A. J., Thornberry, T. P., & Krohn, M. D. (1995). Resilient youth: Identifying factors that prevent high-risk youth from engaging in delinquency and drug use. In J. Hagan (Ed.), *Delinquency and disrepute in the life course* (pp. 217–247). Greenwich, CT: JAI Press.

Smith, G. M., & Fogg, C. P. (1978). Psychological predictors of early use, late use, and nonuse of marijuana among teenage students. In D. B. Kandel (Ed.), *Longitudinal research on drug use* (pp. 101–113). Washington, DC: Hemisphere.

Stack, C. (1974). *All our kin: Strategies for survival in a Black community.* New York: Harper & Row.

Stanley, H., Goldstein, A., & Bry, B. H. (1976). *Program manual for the Early Secondary Intervention Program.* (Available from B. H. Bry, Graduate School of Applied and Professional Psychology, Rutgers University, 152 Frelinghuysen Rd., Piscataway, NJ 08854-8085)

Stephens, D. (1996). Relationship between learned helplessness and urban adolescent problem behavior (Doctoral dissertation, Rutgers University, 1996). *Dissertation Abstracts International, 57,* 7237B.

Sternberg, J., & Bry, B. H. (1994). Solution generation and family conflict over time in problem-solving therapy with families of adolescents: The impact of therapist behavior. *Child & Family Behavior Therapy, 16*(4), 1–23.

Stice, E., Myers, M. G., & Brown, S. A. (1998). A longitudinal grouping analysis of adolescent substance use escalation and de-escalation. *Psychology of Addictive Behaviors, 12,* 14–27.

Straus, M. A., & Sweet, S. (1992). Verbal/symbolic aggression in couples: Incidence rates and relationships to personal characteristics. *Journal of Marriage and the Family, 54,* 346–357.

Streit, F., & Oliver, H. G., Jr. (1972). The child's perception of his family and its relationship to drug use. *Drug Forum, 1,* 283–289.

Sue, D. W., Arredondo, P., & McDavis, R. J. (1992). Multicultural counseling competencies and standards: A call to the profession. *Journal of Counseling and Development, 70*(4), 477–486.

Sue, D. W., & Sue, S. (1990). *Counseling the culturally different.* New York: John Wiley & Sons.

Sue, S., & Zane, N. (1987). The role of culture and cultural techniques in psychotherapy: A critique and reformulation. *American Psychologist, 42*(1), 37–45.

Sue, S., Zane, N., & Young, K. (1994). Research on psychotherapy with culturally diverse populations. In A. E. Bergin & S. L. Garfield (Eds.), *Handbook of psychotherapy and behavior change* (pp. 783–817). New York: John Wiley & Sons.

Swisher, J. D., & Hu, T. W. (1983). Alternatives to drug abuse: Some are and some are not. In T. J. Glynn, C. G. Leukefeld, & J. P. Ludford (Eds.), *Preventing adolescent drug abuse: Intervention strategies* (NIDA Research Monograph No. 47, pp. 141–153). Rockville, MD: National Institute on Drug Abuse.

Tarter, R. E., Alterman, A. I., & Edwards, K. L. (1985). Vulnerability to alcoholism in men: A behavior-genetic perspective. *Journal of Studies on Alcohol, 46*(4), 329–356.

Tatum, J., Moseley, S., Boyd-Franklin, N., & Herzog, E. (1995). A home based family systems approach to the treatment of African American teenage parents and their families. *Zero to Three: Journal of the National Center for Clinical Infant Programs, 15*(4), 18–25.

Taylor, R. D., & Wang, M. C. (Eds.) (1997). *Social and emotional adjustment and family relations in ethnic minority families.* Mahwah, NJ: Erlbaum.

Telleen, S., Herzog, B. S., & Kilbane, T. L. (1989). Impact of a family support program on mothers' social support and parenting stress. *American Journal of Orthopsychiatry, 59*(3), 410–419.

Thomas, E. A. (1995). *Protective factors against substance use in the lives of urban Haitian-American high school students.* Unpublished doctoral dissertation, Rutgers University.

Treadway, D. (1989). *Before it's too late: Working with substance abuse in the family.* New York: Norton.

Tremblay, R. E., Pagani-Kurtz, L., Mosse, L. C., Vitaro, F., & Pihl, R. O. (1995). A bimodal preventive intervention for disruptive kindergarten boys: Its impact through mid-adolescence. *Journal of Consulting and Clinical Psychology, 63,* 560–568.

Trepper, T. S., & Barrett, M. J. (Eds.). (1986). *Treating incest: A multiple systems perspective.* New York: Haworth Press.

Tubman, J. G. (1991). A pilot study of family life among school age children of problem drinking men: Child, mother, and family comparisons. *Family Dynamics of Addiction Quarterly, 1*(1), 10–20.

Turk, E. M. (1993). *Explanatory style and adolescent substance use: A comparison of heavy substance users' and abstainers' spontaneous explanations.* Unpublished doctoral dissertation, Rutgers University.

Turk, E. M., & Bry, B. H. (1992). Adolescents' and parents' explanatory styles and parents' causal explanations about their adolescents. *Cognitive Therapy and Research, 16,* 349–357.

Vaillant, G. E., & Milofsky, E. S. (1982). The etiology of alcoholism: A prospective viewpoint. *American Psychologist, 37*(5), 494–503.

Webster-Stratton, C. (1993). *The incredible years: A trouble-shooting guide for parents of children aged 3–8.* Toronto: Umbrella Press.

Weissbourd, B., & Kagan, S. (1989). Family support programs: Catalysts for change. *American Journal of Orthopsychiatry, 59*(1), 20–31.

Werner, E. E. (1989). Children of the Garden Island. *Scientific American, 260*(4), 106–111.

Wesch, D., & Lutzker, J. R. (1991). A comprehensive 5-year evaluation of Project 12-Ways: An ecobehavioral program for treating and preventing child abuse and neglect. *Journal of Family Violence, 6*(1), 17–35.

Williams, K. (1987). Cultural diversity in family support: Black families. In S. Kagan, D. Powell, B. Weissbourd, & E. Zigler (Eds.), *America's family support programs* (pp. 295–307). New Haven, CT: Yale University Press.

Wills, T. A., Blechman, E. A., & McNamara, G. (1996). Family support, coping, and competence. In E. M. Hetherington & E. A. Blechman (Eds.), *Stress, coping, and resiliency and children and families.* Mahwah, NJ: Erlbaum.

Wolfe, V. V., Gentile, C., Michienzi, T., Sas, L., & Wolfe, D. A. (1991). The children's impact of traumatic events scale: A measure of post-sexual-abuse PTSD symptoms. *Behavioral Assessment, 13,* 359–383.

Zigler, E., & Black, K. (1989). America's family support movement: Strengths and limitations. *American Journal of Orthopsychiatry, 59*(1), 6–19.

Zucker, R. A., Kincaid, S. B., Fitzgerald, H. E., & Bingham, C. R. (1994, August). *Alcohol schema acquisition in preschoolers: Differences between COAs and non-COAs.* Paper presented at the annual meeting of the American Psychological Association, Los Angeles.

Author Index

Subject Index